EAT FAT
LOSE WEIGHT

A GUIDE TO HEALTHY FATS PLUS 70 DELICIOUS RECIPES

pil

Publications International, Ltd.

Publications International, Ltd.

Table of Contents

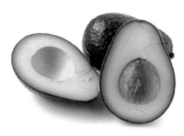
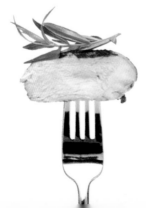
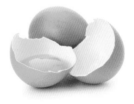

EAT FAT LOSE WEIGHT

DIETARY FATS, WEIGHT AND HEALTH

Want to hear some good news about dietary fats—especially how they relate to weight and health? Eating dietary fats is not as bad as you might think, nor will eating dietary fats necessarily make you fat. The right amounts and types of dietary fats can actually contribute to weight loss and weight maintenance. Fats are essential to your overall diet, and you need to eat fat if you want to lose weight. Understanding what dietary fats are and how they fit into an overall diet will help you with food selection and meal and menu planning.

In addition to their role in weight loss and weight management, different types of dietary fats are important for overall health brain function and longevity.

Dietary fats are naturally found in foods and beverages such as dairy products, eggs, oils, nuts, meats and seeds. Dietary fats are also man-made, found in processed cheeses and meats, margarines and other prepared foods and beverages.

There are differing viewpoints on the benefits of the different types of dietary fats, and the ideal amounts to consume. The purpose of this book is to

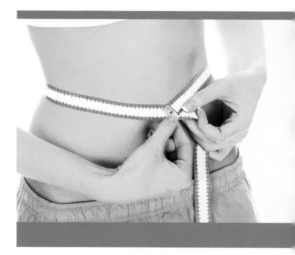

educate you on the types of fats, their contribution to health and to provide recipes that focus on healthy fats, proteins and vegetables, and de-emphasize carbohydrates. Your doctor or registered dietitian/nutritionist can help you determine if this way of eating is appropriate for you.

> *The key, when limiting calorie intake for weight loss, is to choose fats wisely.*

Choose the Right Fats

Contrary to popular belief, we all need some fat in our diets; it's essential for proper body functioning, and it adds flavor to food. But it also provides more than twice the calories of carbohydrate or protein. So the key, when limiting calorie intake for weight loss, is to choose fats wisely. That means cutting way back on harmful saturated fats and replacing them with unsaturated fats.

Types of Fats

Saturated fats are primarily found in foods from animal sources, such as meat, poultry and full-fat dairy products, while trans fats are mostly created when oils are partially hydrogenated to make them better for cooking and to give them a longer shelf life. These fats put you at greater risk for heart disease. Unsaturated fats, on the other hand, are found in plant-based foods (and in some fatty fish, such as salmon, tuna and sardines) and tend to lower your risk of heart problems.

The American Heart Association's (AHA) Nutrition Committee recommends that healthy Americans over 2 years of age consume between 25 and 35 percent of their total daily calories as fats. On a 2,000-calorie diet, this amounts to 500 to 700 calories, or about 56 to 78 grams of fat daily.

They also suggest limiting saturated fat to less than 7 percent of total daily calories. On a 2,000-calorie diet, this is less than 140 calories (only about 16 grams) daily, or the equivalent of about 3 ounces of regular ground beef

(25% fat), 1 ounce of Cheddar cheese (9.4% fat) and 1 cup of whole milk (3.5% fat).

Try to eliminate trans fats (fats that have been processed into saturated fats) completely, or limit them to less than 1 percent of total daily calories. On a 2,000-calorie diet, that means fewer than 20 calories (about 2 grams) should come from trans fats.

What's Inside Fats and Oils?

Fats and oils are composed of fatty acids that contain different properties. Some fatty acids are considered unhealthy and may contribute to certain diseases, while other fatty acids are considered to be healthier and better for weight loss and weight maintenance.

The main types of fatty acids that are found in our food supply include saturated fatty acids, monounsaturated fatty acids, polyunsaturated fatty acids, trans fatty acids, omega-3 and omega-6 fatty acids and triglycerides. Cholesterol is a waxy substance found in foods and beverages, and is also produced by the body.

Saturated fatty acids (or saturated fats) are fully saturated or packed with fatty acids. (The name refers to its chemical makeup; saturated fats are short-chain fats with no double bonds, and are "saturated" with hydrogen.) They are the hardest type of fat for the body to break down and tend to increase the risk for heart disease and stroke.

Saturated fats are mostly found in animal foods such as meats and dairy products and in some tropical oils including coconut, palm and palm kernel oil. By replacing foods and beverages that are high in saturated fatty acids with healthier fatty acids (such as monounsaturated and omega-3 fatty acids), blood cholesterol levels may be lowered and blood profiles may improve.

Monounsaturated fatty acids (or monounsaturated fats) have one space or opening within their chain of fatty acids, which makes it easier for the body to metabolize or break down. Partly for this reason, monounsaturated fats are considered to be healthier than saturated fats. Also, monounsaturated fats may help to lower blood cholesterol.

Monounsaturated fats are found in avocados, canola oil, olives and nuts and their respective oils.

> *Your daily fat consumption should be comprised mostly of monounsaturated or polyunsaturated fats.*

Polyunsaturated fatty acids (or polyunsaturated fats) have many spaces or openings within their chain of fatty acids, which makes them much easier for the body to process.

Polyunsaturated fats may help to reduce blood cholesterol and lower the risk of heart disease and stroke. They also provide nutrients for the development and maintenance of healthy body cells, which include vitamin E, an important antioxidant that protects cells from damage.

Oils with polyunsaturated fats include corn, olive, soybean and sunflower oils. They are liquid at room temperature, but may solidify when chilled.

Polyunsaturated fats can also be found in fatty fish including herring, mackerel, salmon and trout, along with other seafood, nuts and seeds.

Polyunsaturated fats can be beneficial to the heart when consumed in moderation and when they replace saturated and trans fats in the diet. Your daily fat consumption should be comprised mostly of monounsaturated or polyunsaturated fats.

Trans fatty acids (or trans fats) are fatty acids that have been processed into saturated fats. Trans fats are created by industrial methods through the process of hydrogenation, which solidifies or partially solidifies liquid vegetable oils. Trans fats are difficult for the body to process and eliminate. Consequently, trans fats are considered a risk factor in cardiovascular disease.

The terms "hydrogenated" and "partially hydrogenated oils" on the Nutrition Facts Panel typically mean that food contains trans fats. Trans fats are found in many fried foods and baked goods such as crackers, cookies, pastries, pie crust and pizza dough.

In 2015, the U.S. Food and Drug Administration (FDA) determined that partially hydrogenated oils (the primary dietary source of artificial trans fats in processed foods) are "generally not recognized as safe in human food." Food manufacturers were given three years (until 2018) to comply with removing all trans fats from food. Check nutrition labels to make sure you're avoiding all trans fats. Even if a food package states "0 grams of trans fats," it might still contain some trans fats if the amount per serving is less than 0.5 grams, so check the ingredients to make sure there are no hydrogenated or partially hydrogenated oils listed.

Omega-3 and **omega-6 fatty acids** are both types of polyunsaturated fats with unique properties.

Omega-3 fatty acids (or omega-3 fats) are essential fats, which means that they must be supplied by the diet for healthy body functioning. Omega-3 fats, particularly EPA and DHA, are beneficial to the heart. They may decrease arrhythmias (abnormal heartbeats), and triglycerides stored in fat cells, increase tissue flexibility, lower blood pressure,

reduce inflammation and slow the growth of plaque in the arteries. (Plaque is a hard substance that is composed of cholesterol, calcium and clotting materials.)

Good sources of omega-3 fats are seafood such as mackerel, sardines, salmon, tuna and shellfish, and plant sources like walnuts, flaxseed and canola and soybean oils.

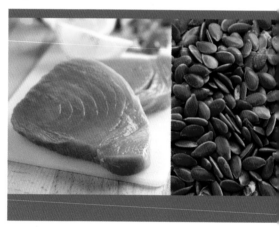

Omega-6 fatty acids (or omega-6 fats) are also polyunsaturated fats and essential fatty acids. Omega-6 fats perform vital roles in brain function, normal growth and development. They also help maintain reproduction, support healthy skin and hair and bone health and regulate metabolism.

However, omega-6 fatty acids may increase inflammation and contribute to complex regional pain syndrome. Chronic inflammation may contribute to asthma, autoimmunity and neurodegenerative diseases, cancers and coronary heart disease.

Omega-6 fats are prevalent in eggs, meats, poultry, salad dressings and corn, grape seed and sunflower oils. They are often used in fried and processed foods, so a diet that is filled with highly processed foods may be disproportionately high in omega-6 fatty acids.

A healthy diet contains a balance of omega-3 and omega-6 fatty acids, although the typical American diet tends to contain more omega-6 fatty acids than omega-3 fatty acids. Consuming more omega-3 fats through food sources may help to balance this pattern.

Cholesterol is a waxy substance that is found in animal foods such as dairy products, eggs and meats. The body also produces cholesterol on its own.

Cholesterol is an essential component in the cell membranes of brain and nerve cells. It is used to maintain brain health for memory formation, and for the production of hormones and vitamin D. When sunlight is absorbed by your skin, cholesterol within the cells is converted to vitamin D.

Common thought used to be that a high level of dietary cholesterol contributed to coronary heart disease, diabetes, stroke or peripheral vascular disease. This is because excess cholesterol can form plaque between the layers of the artery walls. In turn, plaque may clog arteries, reduce their flexibility, interfere with blood circulation and lead to atherosclerosis, or "hardening" of the arteries. Plaque can also break apart and lead to blood clots. If blood clots form and block narrowed arteries, then a heart attack or stroke may occur.

Current thinking focuses more on the type of dietary and blood cholesterol and the types of fatty acids that they transport, and that consuming cholesterol doesn't necessarily lead to higher blood cholesterol levels.

There are two main types of cholesterol: **LDL-cholesterol** (considered to be "bad" cholesterol) and **HDL-cholesterol** (considered to be "good" cholesterol). Too much of one type of cholesterol may place a person at higher risk of coronary heart disease, heart attack, stroke or other conditions.

LDL-cholesterol is considered to be "bad" cholesterol because it contributes to increased plaque in arteries, decreases flexibility and raises the risk of atherosclerosis. Total fat in the diet, dietary cholesterol, saturated fat, trans fats and excess calories are some of the dietary factors that may increase LDL-cholesterol. Lifestyle factors and genetics that may also increase it include age, diabetes, family history, high blood pressure, male gender, obesity and physical inactivity.

HDL-cholesterol is considered to be "good" cholesterol because it helps remove cholesterol from the arteries and transport it back to the liver where it is broken down and excreted from the body. A healthy level of HDL-cholesterol (60 mg/dL or higher) may also protect against heart attack and stroke, while a low level of HDL-cholesterol (less than 40 mg/dL) may increase the risk of heart disease.

The protective benefits of HDL-cholesterol may depend upon the levels of other blood fats that are associated with coronary heart disease. For example, if LDL-cholesterol is not within normal range (100-129 mg/dL), even a high HDL-cholesterol level may not be protective.

Fish and soy foods may increase HDL-cholesterol (good cholesterol), as may moderate

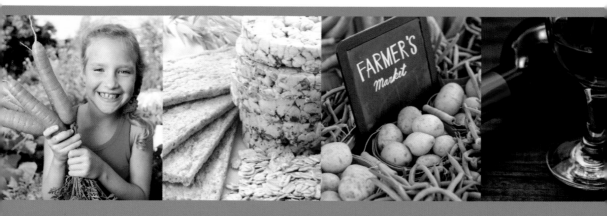

alcohol consumption (red wine in particular). Consuming foods that are high in antioxidants from fruits, vegetables and whole grains may help prevent LDL-cholesterol from injuring the artery walls. Lifestyle factors and genetics that may increase HDL-cholesterol are female gender and physical activity.

Triglycerides are the main form of fat found in food and within the body. Triglycerides are composed of three fatty acids that vary in composition (saturated, unsaturated or a combination). High levels of triglycerides in the blood are associated with atherosclerosis (hardening of the arteries).

Cigarette smoking, excessive alcohol consumption, high carbohydrate intake, overweight and obesity and physical inactivity may all contribute to elevated blood triglycerides.

People with diabetes, heart disease or genetic disorders may also have high blood triglyceride levels. This is because elevated triglycerides are often associated with high blood cholesterol, high LDL-cholesterol and/or low HDL-cholesterol, which are high-risk factors that are connected with these medical conditions.

FAT DIGESTION, ABSORPTION, METABOLISM AND STORAGE

In general, the more solidified the fat or oil, the more difficult it is for the body to process, use, eliminate or store. Avocados, butter, mayonnaise, nut butters, poultry skin and salad dressings have delicious mouth feel due to their composition of fats and oils. From the moment these buttery, creamy, smooth foods are consumed, their complex digestion begins.

Fat Digestion

Fat digestion begins in the mouth, where it is mostly physical. The teeth tear apart fatty foods and the temperature within the mouth melts some of the fats. A gland under the tongue also secretes a fat-splitting enzyme called lipase.

Then the fatty residue passes through the esophagus into the stomach, where it mixes with gastric lipase, an enzyme that is secreted by stomach cells. Gastric lipase continues fat digestion as the stomach muscles churn and mix the stomach contents. Together, this process continues to break down the fat by breaking up large fat molecules into smaller ones and evenly distributing them.

Most of the fats in foods and beverages are packaged in the form of triglycerides, which must be broken down into fatty acids and a molecule called glycerol for absorption. This process tends to be slow. As a result, fats linger in the stomach and contribute to fullness or satiety. This can take up to a few hours and is why a fatty meal is so filling and why a low-fat meal can be so unsatisfying.

Most fat digestion happens after fat passes from the stomach to the small intestine. Once the fatty residue moves inside the small intestine, the smallest fatty acids and glycerol are able to pass through the intestinal wall into the blood. They are transported to the liver where they are converted into energy and other fats as needed. Sometimes the liver stores fat, which is not a healthy condition.

The larger triglycerides are broken down in the small intestine by bile, an emulsifier that is made in the liver and stored in the gallbladder. Bile emulsifies fats by breaking them down with watery digestive secretions and prepares them for additional breakdown by enzymes. The pancreas then secretes a digestive enzyme into the small intestine, which breaks down the emulsified triglycerides even further.

> *Fats linger in the stomach and contribute to fullness or satiety. This can take up to a few hours and is why a fatty meal is so filling and why a low-fat meal can be so unsatisfying.*

Fat Absorption

Fatty acids and cholesterol cannot easily travel in the blood or in the lymph, a watery body fluid that carries the products of fat digestion. This is because they are large molecules, and fat and water do not mix (think oil and vinegar salad dressing that must be shaken before using).

To compensate, fatty acids are packaged inside a protein "shell" for their journey through the bloodstream. These protein packages are called lipoproteins, which means lipids (fats) and protein. The two most well-known types of lipoproteins are low-density lipoproteins (LDL) and high-density lipoproteins (HDL), both discussed in regards to cholesterol on pages 9–10.

HDLs contain the most protein and the least fats and carry cholesterol to the liver for recycling or disposal, while LDLs contain mostly cholesterol. This protein to fat ratio is another reason why HDLs are considered to be "good" and LDLs "bad" for the body.

The fatty acids that are not used by the body are returned to the liver for recycling, disposal or storage. It is easy to see why excess fat in the diet may contribute to greater fat stores. But in certain conditions, fat is converted into energy. All of the body cells can use fatty acids for energy, except for those in the brain, eyes and red blood cells that rely upon glucose.

Fat Metabolism

After dietary fats are digested they can be channeled into energy production. Additionally, enzymes can break down stored fats to release fatty acids into the bloodstream. When these fatty acids reach the muscle cells, they go into the powerhouse of the cell, called the mitochondria.

Fats supply about twice the amount of calories for chemical energy production than carbohydrates or protein: 9 calories per gram for fats compared to 4 calories per gram for both carbohydrates and protein. That is why fats and oils are so calorie (and energy) dense.

In the mitochondria, energy (calories) is removed from the fatty acids that produce chemical energy for metabolism. Carbon dioxide and water are by-products.

Fats supply about twice the amount of calories for chemical energy production than carbohydrates or protein: 9 calories per gram for fats compared to 4 calories per gram for both carbohydrates and protein. That is why fats and oils are so calorie (and energy) dense.

Another type of fat metabolism or breakdown is called ketosis. Ketosis occurs when there is little to no carbohydrates in the diet, which are the body's preferred energy source. Ketosis can occur in prolonged starvation or during high-protein diets that greatly reduce carbohydrate intake. Ketosis utilizes ketones, the by-products of stored fat, rather than carbohydrates (namely glucose) for energy. Diets that are higher in protein and fat and lower in carbohydrates work in a similar manner.

Fat Storage

Fats that are not used by the body are stored in fat cells. Fat cells store small amounts of fat molecules when the concentration of fatty acids in the blood rises, such as after a high-fat meal. An increase in fatty acids in the blood triggers an enzyme called lipase (located in fat tissue) to convert the fatty acids from the blood into a storage form within the fat cells.

The majority of stored fat in the human body is under the skin, called subcutaneous fat. A high percentage of subcutaneous fat surrounds the buttocks, breasts, hips and waist in females. In males, most subcutaneous fat is found around the abdomen, buttocks and chest. There is also fat around the kidneys, liver and inside muscles. A goal in a well-designed diet is to reduce extraneous fat—especially the fat that surrounds the organs and muscles.

During the 1990's when high carbohydrate diets were at their peak in popularity, obesity rates began to rise.

METABOLISM: FAT VERSUS CARBOHYDRATE

Since the 1950's, Americans were advised to reduce fat in their diet for heart disease protection, weight loss and weight maintenance and well-being. Dietary approaches were low in fat and cholesterol and higher in carbohydrates (starches and sugars), while higher protein and fat diets were criticized for supporting rich foods and beverages and contributing to elevated blood cholesterol.

During the 1990's when high carbohydrate diets were at their peak in popularity, obesity rates began to rise. Total calories were implicated in these increases, but also the amounts of carbohydrates in the American diet—particularly processed carbohydrates from refined breadstuffs and sugar-filled beverages—were linked.

Subsequently, new research demonstrated that low-carbohydrate, higher-fat diets actually improve HDL-cholesterol and do not significantly increase LDL-cholesterol. An explanation of carbohydrate metabolism versus fat metabolism explains how this can be possible.

Your body must maintain its blood sugar within a certain range for energy to think, work, exercise and perform other activities. Insulin, a hormone produced by the pancreas, helps to move blood sugar (glucose) into the cells for these functions.

Dietary carbohydrates in the form of starches and sugars supply your body with these needed carbohydrates. The body also has a limited store of glycogen or stored carbohydrates—about 2,500 calories—in reserve that are contained within the muscles, liver and blood. However, this can quickly be used for the increased energy demands of exercise, during fasting and disease states.

In contrast, your body has about 50,000 calories of stored fat with potential energy that it can convert into energy through a complex series of chemical reactions.

After eating or drinking, insulin moves blood sugar into the cells for energy; blood sugar returns to normal levels and you get hungry, eat, and the process repeats. If the pancreas does not produce enough insulin (as in diabetes), this may damage the small blood vessels in the body, and blindness, heart attack, infections, kidney disease, stroke or insufficient wound healing may result. Either oral or injected insulin may be needed.

> *A higher-fat lower-carb diet encourages the body to use ketosis for energy production. This shift in energy metabolism generally results in weight loss.*

If the body runs out of stored carbohydrates, then the liver produces a type of fat known as a ketone that can be converted into energy in a process called ketosis. A higher-fat lower-carb diet encourages the body to use ketosis for energy production, sparing glucose for the brain, eyes and red blood cells. This shift in energy metabolism generally results in weight loss.

Carbohydrates contain water, so part of the initial weight loss in a higher protein and fat and lower carbohydrate diet is the disposal of water stores. Initial weight loss at the beginning may be significant. There may be some temporary side effects such as fatigue, light-headedness or increased urination. It is important to check first with a healthcare provider before beginning a diet of this kind.

Refined carbohydrates (especially those that are low fat) are processed very quickly, first spiking and then crashing blood sugar levels. They're also quite unsatisfying, which can cause you to overeat. Initially the decrease in carbohydrates may be physically and emotionally discomforting, but once the body adjusts to a ketogenic state, more protein and fat in the diet can be satiating. Since fat has twice as many calories per gram as carbohydrates, you may find that you'll be more satisfied with less food.

FAT IN HEALTH AND DISEASE

Fats are essential to the diet and health. Fats function as the body's

> *One of the most important roles of fat in the body is as an energy source, especially when carbohydrates are not available from the diet or are lacking in the body.*

thermostat. The layer of fat just beneath the skin helps to keep the body warm or causes it to sweat to cool the body.

Fat cushions the body from shock, contributes to bile acids, cell membranes and steroid hormones (such as estrogen and testosterone) and helps to regulate fluid balance. Too many or too few fats in the diet may influence each of these important functions.

One of the most important roles of fat in the body is as an energy source, especially when carbohydrates are not available from the diet or are lacking in the body. When people did manual work all day and expended the calories that they consumed, they made good use of carbohydrates and fats in their diet and within their energy stores. Today's laborsaving devices and sedentary lifestyles create less need for excess carbohydrate and

fat calories, no matter if they are from animal or plant sources.

Over the years, as we moved from a plant-based diet toward an animal-based diet, the composition of fatty acids in the American diet switched from monounsaturated and polyunsaturated fats to more saturated fats, which are associated more with cardiovascular disease. Incorporating more plant-based foods and beverages into your diet helps supports a healthier proportion of fats in the body for weight maintenance and good health.

Besides cardiovascular disease, excess saturated and trans fats in the diet are associated with certain cancers, cerebral vascular disease, diabetes, obesity and metabolic syndrome (a collection of conditions that may include abnormal cholesterol or triglyceride levels, excess body fat around the waist, high blood sugar and increased blood pressure that may increase one's risk of diabetes, heart disease and/or stroke.

The Cholesterol Controversy

Atherosclerosis, or hardening of the arteries, is not a modern disease. Rather, the correlation between blood cholesterol and cardiovascular disease was recognized as far back as the 1850's.

One hundred years later in the 1950's, cholesterol and saturated fats in the diet were implicated as major risk factors for cardiovascular disease. Then in the 1980's, major U.S. health institutions determined that the process of lowering blood cholesterol (specifically LDL-cholesterol) reduces the risk of heart attacks that are caused by coronary heart disease.

Some scientists questioned this conclusion, marking the unofficial start of what's been called the "cholesterol controversy". Studies of cholesterol-lowering drugs known as statins supported the idea that reducing blood cholesterol means less mortality from heart disease. Subsequent statin studies have questioned this association. Other factors aside from dietary cholesterol have since been identified that may lead to elevated blood cholesterol, such as trans fats.

The liver manufactures cholesterol, so reducing cholesterol in the diet *should* help reduce blood cholesterol, coronary heart disease and the risk of heart attack. But in some individuals the liver produces more cholesterol than the body requires and cardiovascular disease can still develop. So dietary cholesterol does not necessarily predict cardiovascular disease or a heart attack.

While dietary cholesterol can be a measure for greater risk, cardiovascular disease and heart attacks are also dependent on such lifestyle and genetic factors as age, diet, exercise, gender, genetics, medication and stress. Reducing hydrogenated fats, saturated fats, total fat and trans fats; incorporating mono- and polyunsaturated fats, switching to more of a plant-based diet and losing weight to help better manage blood fats are other sensible measures to take.

Longer-term weight management is also a preventative measure in cardiovascular disease. Reducing total fat, saturated fat and cholesterol in the diet while increasing consumption of plant-based foods with mono- and polyunsaturated fats and oils, dietary fiber, antioxidants and other phytonutrients can lead to a decrease in overall calorie consumption.

SO WHAT (AND HOW) SHOULD I EAT?

If you want to lose fat, you need to take in fewer calories than you burn. There's simply no getting around this fact. If you're an average woman over 40, restricting your caloric intake can be a good starting point. If you are of shorter stature and/or very inactive, or you haven't dropped any pounds after a couple of weeks at this level, consider lowering that daily intake in 100-calorie increments until you start seeing the weight come off. But don't go much below 1,000 without your doctor's supervision. (And be sure to check with your

doctor before making major changes to your diet or activity level, especially if you have any serious health problems.) The recipes in this book are designed to fit nicely into this lower-calorie eating plan.

If you want to lose fat, you need to take in fewer calories than you burn. There's simply no getting around this fact.

In order to make room for healthy fats without busting your calorie budget, you will have to give up hefty portions of fatty meats. You don't want to skimp on protein, though, because it helps you maintain and build calorie-burning muscle and keeps you feeling full between meals. So select smaller amounts (about 3 ounces) of lean meat and poultry or protein sources that also supply monounsaturated fats and other heart-healthy unsaturated fats; good options include nuts and seeds, dried beans and peas, lentils and fish. (Fatty fish, such as salmon, tuna, trout, mackerel and herring, are rich in good-for-you polyunsaturated fats, especially disease-fighting omega-3s). You'll also need to replace highly processed foods full of saturated and trans fats, sugar and refined carbohydrates with minimally processed fiber- and nutrient-rich vegetables, fruits and grains. What you'll end up with is a nutrient-dense, healthy, satisfying eating plan that's low enough in calories for you to lose weight. It's a plan that will help you shed excess pounds, and you should continue even after you've lost the weight so that it doesn't come back.

If you've ever tried to lose weight before, you know how quickly between-meal hunger can sabotage your best efforts. When your stomach starts growling hours before your next meal, it's incredibly tempting to grab whatever is available. Often, that "whatever" is some unhealthy packaged snack food loaded with sugar, bad fats, sodium and empty calories. Or, if you manage to ignore that hunger, you end up so ravenous at the next meal that you gobble down far more calories than your body actually needs.

Don't skimp on protein, though, because it helps you maintain and build calorie-burning muscle and keeps you feeling full between meals.

To prevent hunger from foiling your weight-loss efforts, don't go more than four (waking) hours without a meal or snack. Every day, have three balanced, 400- to 500-calorie meals, including a source of protein, vegetables or fruit and unsaturated fat. You can also include small amounts of carbohydrate in the form of whole grains. The remainder of your calorie budget for the day should go toward one or two planned snacks, each one including some hunger-fighting protein, a "good fat" like nuts, and veggies, fruit and/or whole grains. An easy, portable snack might include celery sticks, apple slices or a few whole wheat crackers spread with a little almond butter.

Foods for Healthy Living

vegetables and fruit
- apples
- asparagus
- avocados
- bell peppers
- berries
- broccoli
- cabbage
- carrots
- cauliflower
- chard
- citrus
- eggplant
- garlic
- grapes
- green beans
- herbs, fresh
- kale
- mushrooms
- onions
- peaches
- plums
- spinach
- tomatoes
- zucchini

lean meats, grass-fed and organic
- beef, grass-fed
- lamb, grass-fed
- pork, lean cuts
- pork tenderloin
- poultry, organic
- veal chops

seafood, sustainably-farmed
- anchovies
- clams
- crab
- herring
- lobster
- oysters
- salmon
- sardines
- scallops
- shrimp
- tuna

other proteins, fats and oils
- coconut oil
- eggs
- nuts, unsalted roasted
- nut butters, unsweetened
- nut milk
- nut oils
- olive oil
- seeds (chia, flax, pumpkin, sunflower)
- tofu, organic

dairy and nondairy
- clarified butter and ghee
- cottage cheese
- nondairy milk
- soymilk

pantry staples
- almond flour
- coconut flour
- coffee and tea
- dark chocolate
- dried herbs and spices
- mustard
- vinegar

Foods to Consume in Moderation

starchy vegetables
- beets
- butternut squash
- sweet potatoes

whole grains and legumes
- quinoa
- brown rice
- buckwheat
- beans
- legumes

low-fat dairy
- cheese, part-skim
- goat cheese
- Greek yogurt, low-fat
- milk, low-fat
- plain yogurt, low-fat
- ricotta, part-skim

Foods to Limit or Avoid

high-fat proteins
- corned beef
- fried fish
- hot dogs
- lunch meats like bologna and salami
- pork sausage
- ribs

high-fat dairy
- full-fat dairy
- full-fat cheeses
- lard
- margarine

refined carbohydrates
- bread
- pasta
- sugar
- sugar-laden beverages
- sugar substitutes
- white flour

NOTES ON RECIPES AND INGREDIENTS

Since eggs are no longer an issue vis-à-vis cholesterol, they are used freely through the recipes, particularly in the breakfast section. You'll find frittatas, omelets and scrambled eggs, with healthy-fat accompaniments like avocado, goat cheese and turkey sausage.

For snacks, there are deviled eggs and high-protein egg white salad, in addition to healthy nut mixes that include almonds, cashews and pine nuts.

Salads feature avocado, beef, chicken, feta and goat cheese, salmon, tofu, tuna and walnuts with dressings made from healthy oils that include mustard dressing and cranberry and strawberry vinaigrettes.

Soups are protein-based and made with healthy fats. These include fish soups such as Salmon and Wild Rice Chowder and Shrimp Gazpacho; chicken soups such as Chunky Chicken Stew and turkey soups such as Turkey Albondigas Soup.

The meat and seafood recipes showcase a variety of healthy-fat proteins that include beef pot roast, braised chicken, chicken burgers, flank steak, ginger beef, ground beef, chicken and lamb. In the fish and seafood chapter, crab, halibut, mahimahi, mussels, orange roughy, salmon, scallops, scrod, shrimp, tilapia and trout are baked, blackened, broiled, grilled, marinated, pan-seared, seared, stuffed and prepared as kabobs or in parchment.

Side dishes include caramelized vegetables, "chips" and gratins with antioxidant-rich vegetables and heart-healthy grains.

What's a diet without some fun? You'll discover delicious fruit and vegetable smoothies and whips among the final recipes to have as mini-meals, snacks or to enhance lower-fat and lower-calorie meals.

The verdict on many fat-containing foods and beverages is constantly changing. Just when you think something is good or "safe" to consume, some potentially incriminating information is released that questions the validity.

As a result, some foods and beverages have been scrutinized for their efficacy in a healthy diet. These include (but are not limited to) avocados, butter and margarine, cheese, chocolate, coconut, coconut milk and coconut oil, nuts and seeds and oils.

Avocados

Avocados do have a lot of fat, but don't avoid them because of it! They contain omega-3 fatty acids, protein and fiber, as well as the B-vitamins, vitamin C, E and K, magnesium, potassium and healthy monounsaturated fatty acids. One cup of sliced avocado contains about 234 calories, 21 grams of total fat, 3.1 grams of saturated fat, 14 grams of monounsaturated fat and 2.7 grams of polyunsaturated fat with no cholesterol.

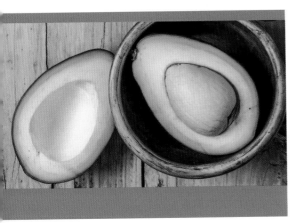

Butter and Margarine

You might be confused about what to think about butter and margarine; there has been a lot of debate and controversy about which you should use. Both have their limitations. Where you would use butter or margarine, choose olive oil (for finishing and serving) or vegetable oil (for cooking). Or use ghee (clarified butter). If a substitution doesn't work, butter is okay in limited quantities, but limit margarine.

Butter has both short and medium "chain" fatty acids. The short chain is called butyric acid and the medium chain is called myristic acid. Both of these saturated fats have healthy benefits. They are relatively easy to transport and absorb by the body and they help supply flavor. In comparison, stearic and palmitic acids, the longer chain fatty acids found in butter, may be cardiovascular risk factors in higher amounts in the diet.

Cheese

Use cheese sparingly in small amounts to add taste, texture and healthy fats to recipes.

Chocolate

The fat that is found in cocoa plants and predominant in dark chocolate is cocoa butter, which is about 33 percent monounsaturated oleic fatty acid and 33 percent stearic fatty acid. In general, stearic fatty acids from plants, although saturated, seem to neither lower high HDL-cholesterol nor increase LDL- or total cholesterol.

Coconut, Coconut Milk and Coconut Oil

Coconut and coconut oil are used throughout the world for their distinctive tastes and textures. Both were considered unhealthy due to their saturated fat content but are now valued for their healthful properties.

Natural cholesterol-free coconut oil can be substituted for cholesterol-containing butter or lard in cooking and baking. It is solid at room temperature but turns liquid at relatively low temperatures about (80°F). The two main types available are refined and virgin; both are acceptable for cooking and baking, but virgin coconut oil has more a coconutty flavor than refined.

There are many liquid coconut products available; they cannot generally be used interchangeably. Coconut milk is made by simmering shredded coconut in water and then straining out and squeezing the coconut to extract the liquid. Coconut water is the liquid from the inside of a coconut and is sold for drinking, not cooking. Coconut milk beverages act as a milk substitute. Coconut cream is similar to coconut milk, but is thicker because it contains less water. Often a layer of coconut cream will separate from the milk in a can of regular coconut milk. To blend it back into the milk, shake the can before opening. Or just dump the whole can into whatever you're cooking and stir well (the heat will melt the cream back into the milk). Avoid cream of coconut; this is sweetened coconut cream and it used primarily in desserts and drinks.

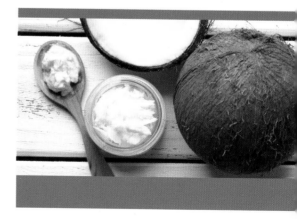

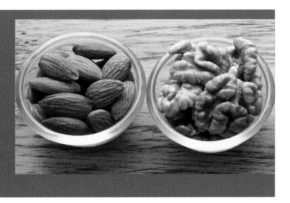

The fatty acids in almonds and walnuts may actually be helpful in lowering other blood fats.

Nuts and Seeds

Nuts and seeds range in total fat, fatty acids and other nutrients. They are filled with protein, mostly mono-and polyunsaturated fatty acids and omega-3 fatty acids, insoluble fiber, the B vitamins and vitamin E, and magnesium, manganese, phosphorus and zinc among other nutrients.

The fatty acids in almonds and walnuts may actually be helpful in lowering other blood fats. Additionally, many nuts have a low Glycemic Index (GI) value, which means that they are useful in insulin management and a good snack.

Pine nuts, common to heart-healthy Mediterranean diets, add a distinctive buttery and creamy touch to recipes. One-half cup contains about

673 calories, 10 grams of protein, 78 grams of total fat, 7 grams of saturated fat, almost 45 grams of monounsaturated fat, 24 grams of polyunsaturated fat and no cholesterol. The amount of dietary fiber ranges from 7 to 12 grams per half cup.

Oils

Like butter and margarine, some oils are also controversial—particularly the tropical oils: coconut oil, palm oil and palm kernel oil. Palm oil is an all-purpose cooking oil that is used in vegetable oil blends to impart flavor. It contains about 51 percent saturated fat, 39 percent monounsaturated fat and 10 percent polyunsaturated fat. Palm kernel oil contains about 86 percent saturated fat, 12 percent monounsaturated fat and 2 percent polyunsaturated fat.

In contrast, canola oil, olive oil and peanut oil have more favorable fatty acid profiles. Canola oil contains about 6 percent saturated fatty acids, 62 percent monounsaturated fatty acids and 32 percent polyunsaturated fatty acids. It is commonly used for baking, frying and in salad dressings.

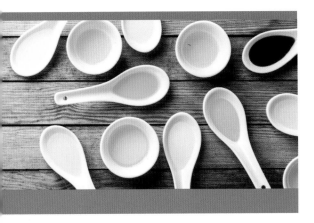

Olive oil contains about 14 percent saturated fatty acids, 73 percent monounsaturated fatty acids and 11 percent polyunsaturated fatty acids. Extra virgin olive oil is primarily used to dress salads, vegetables and entrées. Virgin olive oil is used as an all-purpose cooking oil and in salad dressing. Light and extra-light olive oil generally have less flavor and are primarily used for sautéing and stir-frying since they can withstand more heat than extra virgin olive oil.

Peanut oil contains about 18 percent saturated fatty acids, 49 percent monounsaturated fatty acids and 33 percent polyunsaturated fatty acids. Peanut oil has a higher smoke point than most olive oil blends, so is useful as an all-purpose oil in cooking, frying and in margarines and salad dressings. Peanut oil is commonly used in Asian cuisine; olive oil in Mediterranean cuisine and canola oil tends to cross cuisines in cooking applications.

THE FUTURE OF DIETING

Past and current dietary imperatives have ranged from plant-based to animal-based diets, with and without grains, nuts and seeds, fish and seafood, vegetables and fruits and fats and oils. Processed foods and beverages have permeated our diets with calories, sugars and sodium.

For every research study that has supported favorable foods, beverages and dietary approaches, other studies negate findings and advocate other directives. What is the best diet? Dietary advice? What are the best foods and beverages to consume today or for future health and wellness?

A food scientist's laboratory looks much different than a farmer's field. It is filled with the newest ingredients to create foods and beverages that look, feel, taste and smell much different than we now know or can conceive. In contrast, a farmer's field yields vegetables, fruits, grains and protein-rich foods for field-to-plate freshness, flavor, eating enjoyment and health. In may not be conceivable to eat exclusively one way or the other.

> *Your best approach should be to eat foods in moderation, balance your choices and enjoy a variety of heathy foods.*

What will the optimal diet look like in the future? Will it be test tube-based, farm derived, or some combination of both ideologies? What will be the optimal amounts of protein, fats and carbohydrates? Will there be a universal approach to dieting, or will it be individually based? How will activity be accounted for, or will foods and beverages take this factor (and genetics) into consideration?

This is all difficult to speculate. We do know that dieting is more than numbers—it is the sum of all of the factors that involve what we consume and where and how we do it that matter. Food is more than calories or nutrients—it nourishes our enjoyment and well being. It is a treat to the senses and the soul. There are always going to be new diets—both fad diets and healthy diets. Your best approach should be to eat foods in moderation, balance your choices and enjoy a variety of heathy foods.

The recipes in this book demonstrate that food can be good to eat and good for you, too. You can eat fat and lose weight. Eat healthy fats in moderation with leaner proteins, healthier carbs and plenty of vegetables and fruits in the right proportions to lose weight tastefully and healthfully.

BREAKFAST

ZUCCHINI AND DILL OMELET

4 egg whites

1 egg

2 tablespoons milk

½ teaspoon dried dill
  weed

⅛ teaspoon salt

⅛ teaspoon black
  pepper

1 teaspoon butter

1 cup diced zucchini

1. Whisk egg whites, eggs, milk, dill, salt and pepper in medium bowl until blended.

2. Spray medium skillet with nonstick cooking spray. Add butter; melt over medium-high heat. Add zucchini; cook 4 minutes or until lightly browned, stirring occasionally.

3. Add egg mixture; cook until edges are set. Gently lift edge of egg mixture, allowing uncooked portion to flow underneath. When eggs are set, fold omelet over. Cut in half to serve.

MAKES 2 SERVINGS

Calories 100, Total Fat 5g, Saturated Fat 2g, Cholesterol 111mg, Sodium 290mg, Carbohydrates 3g, Dietary Fiber 1g, Protein 12g

VEGETABLE FRITTATA

1 teaspoon canola oil

1 clove garlic, minced

¼ cup chopped onion

¾ cup chopped broccoli

¼ cup chopped mushrooms

½ cup chopped fresh spinach

4 egg whites

⅛ teaspoon salt

Black pepper

2 tablespoons shredded Cheddar, Parmesan or Monterey Jack cheese

1. Preheat broiler. Heat oil in small nonstick ovenproof skillet over medium-high heat. Add garlic and onion; cook and stir 1 minute. Stir in broccoli and mushrooms; cook, covered, over medium heat just until vegetables are tender. Stir in spinach.

2. Whisk egg whites, salt and pepper in small bowl until well blended.

3. Pour egg whites over vegetables in skillet; cook until egg whites are firm but top is slightly moist. Sprinkle with cheese; broil about 2 minutes or until egg whites are cooked through and cheese is melted.

MAKES 2 SERVINGS

Calories 108, Total Fat 5g, Saturated Fat 2g, Cholesterol 7mg, Sodium 322mg, Carbohydrates 6g, Dietary Fiber 1g, Protein 11g

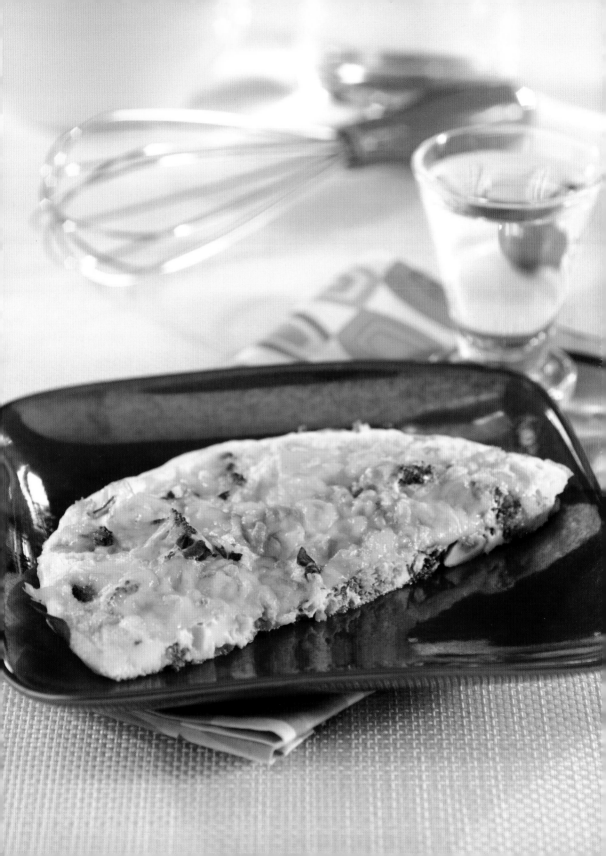

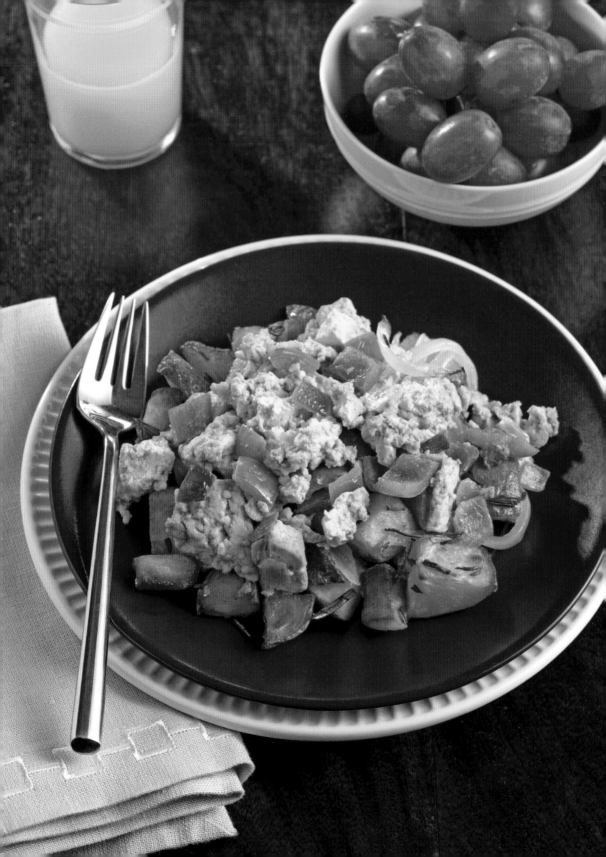

SCRAMBLED TOFU AND POTATOES

POTATOES

- ¼ cup olive oil
- 4 red potatoes, cubed
- ½ white onion, sliced
- 1 tablespoon chopped fresh rosemary
- 1 teaspoon coarse salt

SCRAMBLED TOFU

- ¼ cup nutritional yeast
- ½ teaspoon ground turmeric
- 2 tablespoons water
- 2 tablespoons soy sauce
- 1 package (14 ounces) firm tofu
- 2 teaspoons olive oil
- ½ cup chopped green bell pepper
- ½ cup chopped red onion

1. For potatoes, preheat oven to 450°F. Add ¼ cup olive oil to 12-inch cast-iron skillet; place skillet in oven 10 minutes to heat.

2. Bring large saucepan of water to a boil. Add potatoes; cook 5 to 7 minutes or until tender. Drain and return to saucepan; stir in white onion, rosemary and salt. Spread mixture in preheated skillet. Bake 25 to 30 minutes or until potatoes are browned, stirring every 10 minutes.

3. For tofu, combine nutritional yeast and turmeric in small bowl. Stir in water and soy sauce until smooth.

4. Cut tofu into large cubes. Gently squeeze out water; loosely crumble tofu into medium bowl. Heat 2 teaspoons olive oil in large skillet over medium-high heat. Add bell pepper and red onion; cook and stir 2 minutes or until soft but not browned. Add tofu; drizzle with 3 tablespoons nutritional yeast sauce. Cook and stir about 5 minutes or until liquid is evaporated and tofu is heated through. Stir in additional sauce for stronger flavor, if desired.

5. Divide potatoes among four serving plates; top with tofu.

MAKES 4 SERVINGS

Calories 357, Total Fat 13g, Saturated Fat 3g, Cholesterol 0mg, Sodium 1176mg, Carbohydrates 43g, Dietary Fiber 6g, Protein 15g

PEA AND SPINACH FRITTATA

1 cup chopped onion

¼ cup water

1 cup frozen peas

1 cup fresh spinach

6 egg whites

2 eggs

½ cup cooked brown rice

¼ cup milk

2 tablespoons grated Romano or Parmesan cheese, plus additional for garnish

1 tablespoon chopped fresh mint *or* 1 teaspoon dried mint

¼ teaspoon black pepper

⅛ teaspoon salt

1. Spray large skillet with nonstick cooking spray. Combine onion and water in skillet. Bring to a boil over high heat. Reduce heat to medium; cover and cook 2 to 3 minutes or until onion is tender. Stir in peas; cook until heated through. Drain. Add spinach; cook and stir 1 minute or until spinach just begins to wilt.

2. Combine egg whites, eggs, rice, milk, 2 tablespoons cheese, mint, pepper and salt in medium bowl.

3. Add egg mixture to skillet. Cook without stirring 2 minutes or until eggs begin to set. Gently lift edge of egg mixture, allowing uncooked portion to flow underneath. Remove skillet from heat when eggs are almost set but surface is still moist.

4. Cover and let stand 3 to 4 minutes or until surface is set. Sprinkle with additional cheese, if desired. Cut into four wedges to serve.

MAKES 4 SERVINGS

Calories 162, **Total Fat** 4g, **Saturated Fat** 1g, **Cholesterol** 110mg, **Sodium** 246mg, **Carbohydrates** 18g, **Dietary Fiber** 4g, **Protein** 14g

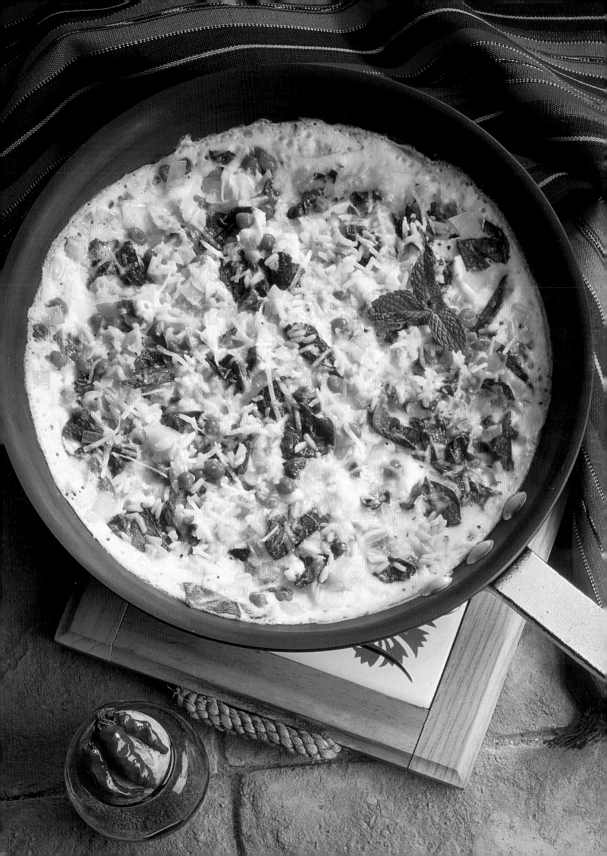

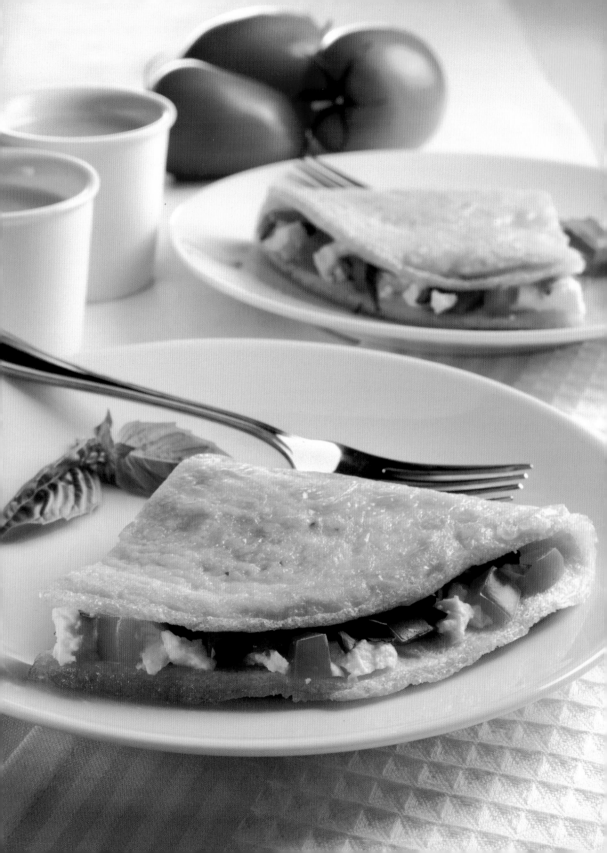

GOAT CHEESE AND TOMATO OMELET

3 egg whites

2 eggs

1 tablespoon water

⅛ teaspoon salt

⅛ teaspoon black pepper

⅓ cup crumbled goat cheese

1 medium plum tomato, diced

2 tablespoons chopped fresh basil or parsley

1. Whisk egg whites, eggs, water, salt and pepper in medium bowl.

2. Spray medium nonstick skillet with nonstick cooking spray; heat over medium heat. Add egg mixture; cook 2 minutes or until eggs begin to set on bottom. Lift edge of omelet to allow uncooked portion of eggs to flow underneath. Cook 3 minutes or until center is almost set.

3. Sprinkle cheese, tomato and basil in center of omelet. Fold half of omelet over filling. Cook 1 to 2 minutes or until cheese begins to melt and center is set. Cut omelet in half; transfer to serving plates.

MAKES 2 SERVINGS

Calories 80, Total Fat 5g, Saturated Fat 3g, Cholesterol 63mg, Sodium 239mg, Carbohydrates 2g, Dietary Fiber 0g, Protein 8g

SWEET POTATO AND TURKEY SAUSAGE HASH

1 turkey Italian sausage link (about 4 ounces)

1 small red onion, finely chopped

1 small red bell pepper, finely chopped

1 small sweet potato, peeled and cut into ½-inch cubes

¼ teaspoon salt (optional)

¼ teaspoon black pepper

⅛ teaspoon ground cumin

⅛ teaspoon chipotle chili powder

1. Remove sausage from casings. Shape sausage into ½-inch balls. Spray large nonstick skillet with nonstick cooking spray; heat over medium heat. Add sausage; cook and stir 3 to 5 minutes or until browned. Remove from skillet; set aside.

2. Spray same skillet with cooking spray. Add onion, bell pepper, sweet potato, salt, if desired, black pepper, cumin and chili powder; cook and stir 5 to 8 minutes or until sweet potato is tender.

3. Stir in sausage; cook without stirring 5 minutes or until hash is lightly browned.

MAKES 2 SERVINGS

Calories 186, Total Fat 4g, Saturated Fat 1g, Cholesterol 17mg, Sodium 417mg, Carbohydrates 23g, Dietary Fiber 4g, Protein 13g

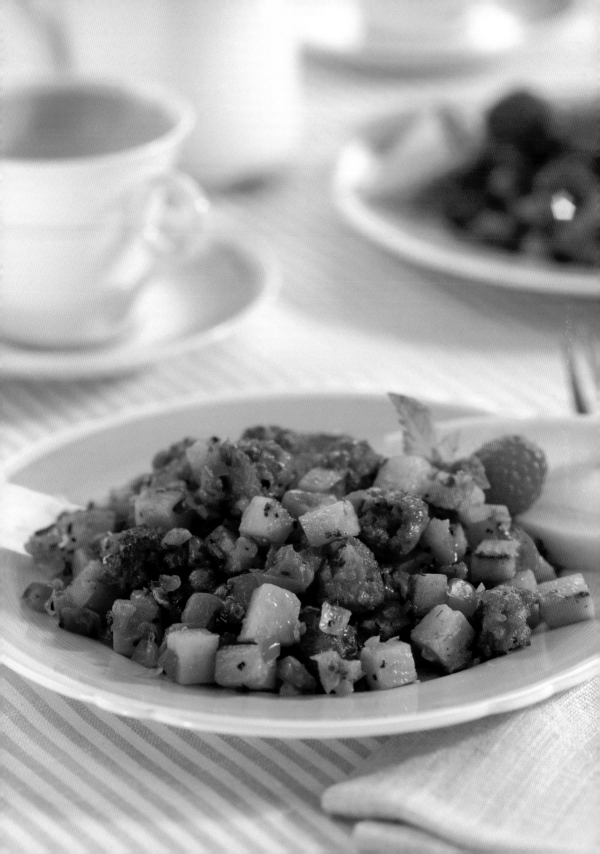

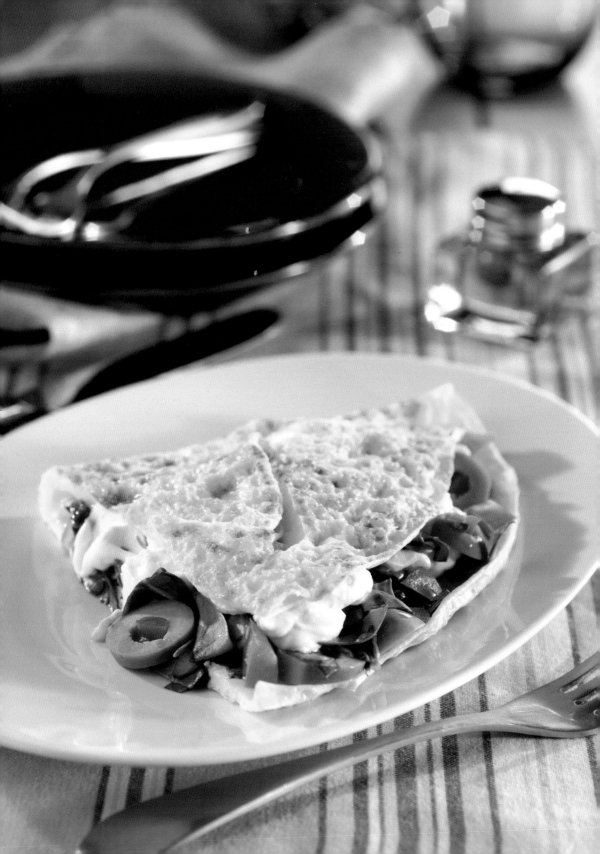

SPINACH, PEPPER AND OLIVE OMELET

1 cup diced red bell pepper

½ teaspoon dried rosemary

⅛ teaspoon red pepper flakes

2 cups loosely packed baby spinach, coarsely chopped

16 stuffed green olives, such as manzanilla, coarsely chopped

2 tablespoons chopped fresh basil

Salt and black pepper

8 eggs

3 tablespoons milk

2 ounces crumbled goat cheese, divided

1. Spray medium skillet with nonstick cooking spray; heat over medium-high heat. Add bell pepper, rosemary and red pepper flakes; cook 4 minutes or until soft, stirring frequently. Stir in spinach; cook until spinach is slightly wilted. Stir in olives and basil. Transfer to medium bowl; season with salt and black pepper.

2. Whisk eggs and milk in large bowl until well blended. Wipe skillet clean with damp paper towel. Coat skillet with cooking spray and heat over medium heat. Add half of egg mixture; cook 2 minutes or until eggs begin to set on bottom. Lift edge of omelet to allow uncooked portion of eggs to flow underneath.

3. When egg mixture is set, spoon half of spinach mixture over half of omelet. Top with half of cheese; fold omelet in half. Slide omelet onto serving plate and cover with foil to keep warm. Repeat with remaining ingredients to make second omelet. Cut omelets in half to serve.

MAKES 4 SERVINGS

Calories 230, Total Fat 15g, Saturated Fat 6g, Cholesterol 390mg, Sodium 570mg, Carbohydrates 5g, Dietary Fiber 2g, Protein 17g

EDAMAME FRITTATA

2 tablespoons olive oil

½ cup frozen shelled edamame

⅓ cup frozen corn

1 shallot, chopped

5 eggs

¾ teaspoon dried Italian seasoning

½ teaspoon salt

½ teaspoon black pepper

4 green onions, chopped

½ cup crumbled goat cheese

1. Preheat broiler. Heat oil in large broilerproof skillet over medium-high heat. Add edamame, corn and shallot; cook and stir 6 to 8 minutes or until shallot is browned and edamame are hot.

2. Meanwhile, whisk eggs, Italian seasoning, salt and pepper in medium bowl. Stir in green onions. Pour egg mixture over vegetables in skillet. Sprinkle with cheese. Cook over medium heat 5 to 7 minutes or until eggs are set on bottom, lifting edge of frittata to allow uncooked portion to flow underneath.

3. Broil 6 inches from heat 1 minute or until top is puffy and golden. Loosen frittata from skillet with spatula; slide onto small plate. Cut into wedges.

MAKES 4 SERVINGS

Calories 240, Total Fat 18g, Saturated Fat 5g, Cholesterol 250mg, Sodium 460g, Carbohydrates 8g, Dietary Fiber 2g, Protein 13g

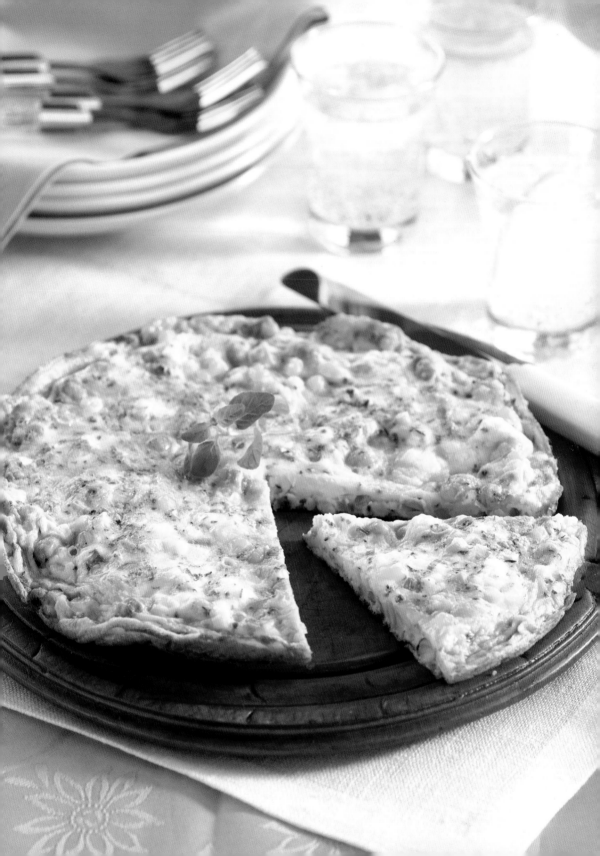

TOMATO OMELET WITH AVOCADO

6 ounces plum tomatoes, chopped (about 1½ tomatoes)

2 to 4 tablespoons chopped fresh cilantro

¼ teaspoon salt

8 eggs

¼ cup soymilk

1 ripe medium avocado, diced

1 small cucumber, chopped

1. Preheat oven to 200°F. Combine tomatoes, cilantro and salt in small bowl; set aside.

2. Whisk eggs and soymilk in medium bowl until well blended.

3. Heat small nonstick ovenproof skillet over medium heat; coat with cooking spray. Pour half of egg mixture into skillet; cook 2 minutes or until eggs begin to set. Lift edge of omelet to allow uncooked portion to flow underneath. Cook 3 minutes or until set.

4. Spoon half of tomato mixture over half of omelet. Loosen omelet with spatula and fold in half. Slide omelet onto serving plate and keep warm in oven. Repeat with remaining ingredients to make second omelet. Cut omelets in half; top with avocado and cucumber.

MAKES 4 SERVINGS

Calories 250, **Total Fat** 17g, **Saturated Fat** 4g, **Cholesterol** 370mg, **Sodium** 300mg, **Carbohydrates** 11g, **Dietary Fiber** 5g, **Protein** 15g

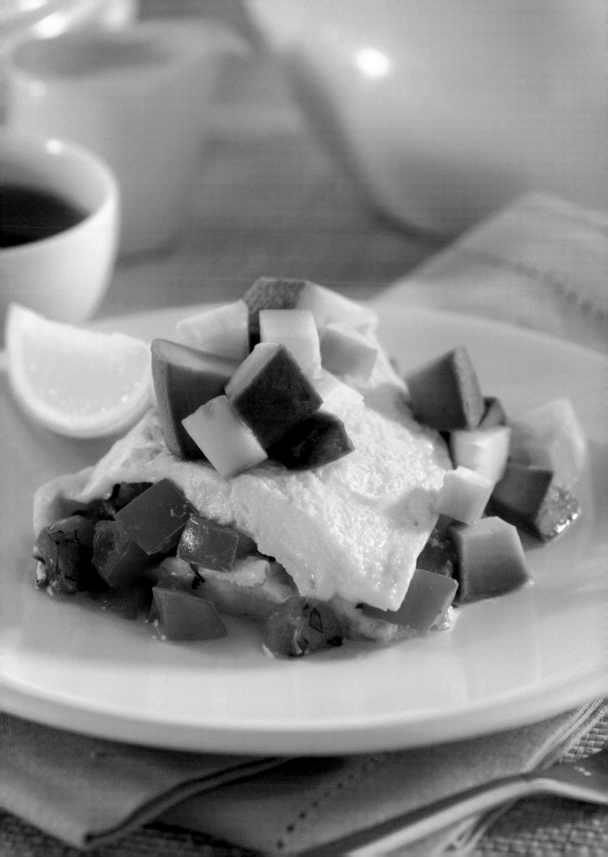

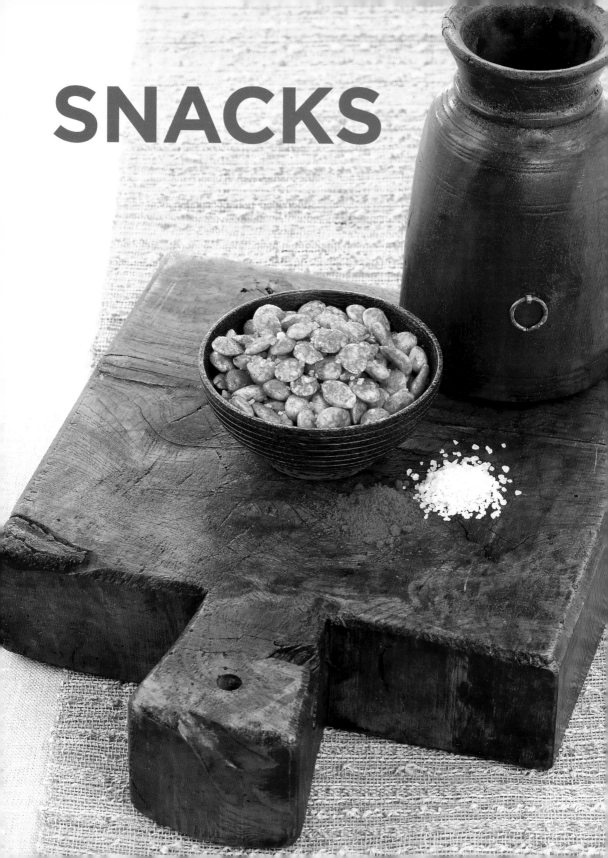

SNACKS

PAPRIKA–SPICED ALMONDS

1 cup whole blanched
  almonds

1 teaspoon olive oil

¼ teaspoon coarse
  salt

¼ teaspoon smoked
  paprika or paprika

1. Preheat oven to 375°F. Spread almonds in single layer in shallow baking pan. Bake 8 to 10 minutes or until almonds are lightly browned. Transfer to bowl; cool 5 to 10 minutes.

2. Drizzle oil over almonds; stir to coat. Sprinkle with salt and paprika; mix well.

MAKES ABOUT 8 SERVINGS

Tip: *For the best flavor, serve these almonds the day they are made.*

Calories 110, **Total Fat** 10g, **Saturated Fat** 1g, **Cholesterol** 0mg, **Sodium** 60mg, **Carbohydrates** 4g, **Dietary Fiber** 2g, **Protein** 4g

GRILLED EGGPLANT ROLL-UPS

4 eggplant slices
   (1 inch thick)

½ teaspoon salt

   Olive oil

4 tablespoons
   hummus

¼ cup crumbled feta
   cheese

¼ cup chopped green
   onions

4 tomato slices

1. Lay eggplant slices on wire rack set over baking sheet. Sprinkle with salt; let stand 15 minutes.

2. Prepare grill for direct cooking. Lightly brush eggplant with olive oil. Grill over medium-high heat 10 minutes; turn and brush with olive oil. Grill 10 minutes or until tender. Let stand until cool enough to handle.

3. Spread 1 tablespoon hummus on each eggplant slice. Top with feta, green onions and tomato. Roll up tightly. Serve immediately.

MAKES 2 SERVINGS

Calories 96, Total Fat 6g, Saturated Fat 4g, Cholesterol 25mg, Sodium 326mg, Carbohydrates 5g, Dietary Fiber 1g, Protein 5g

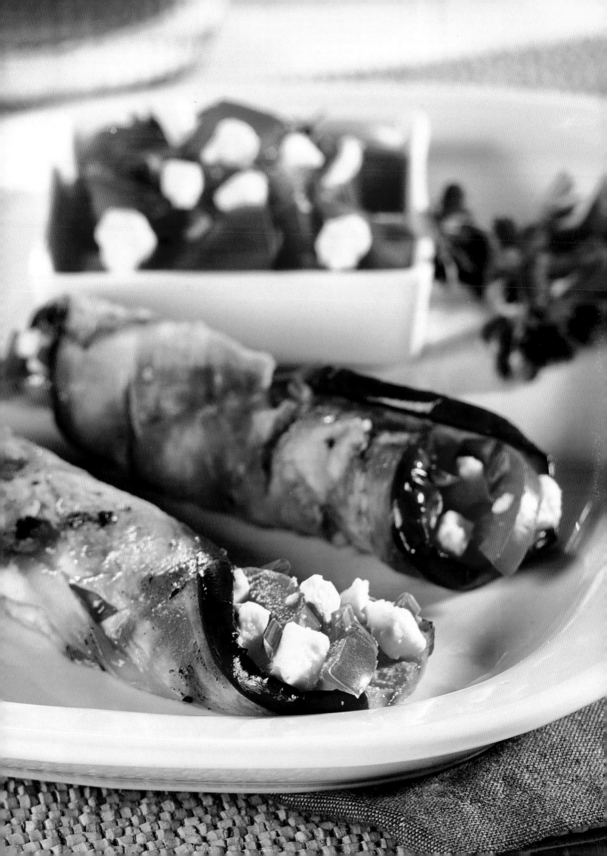

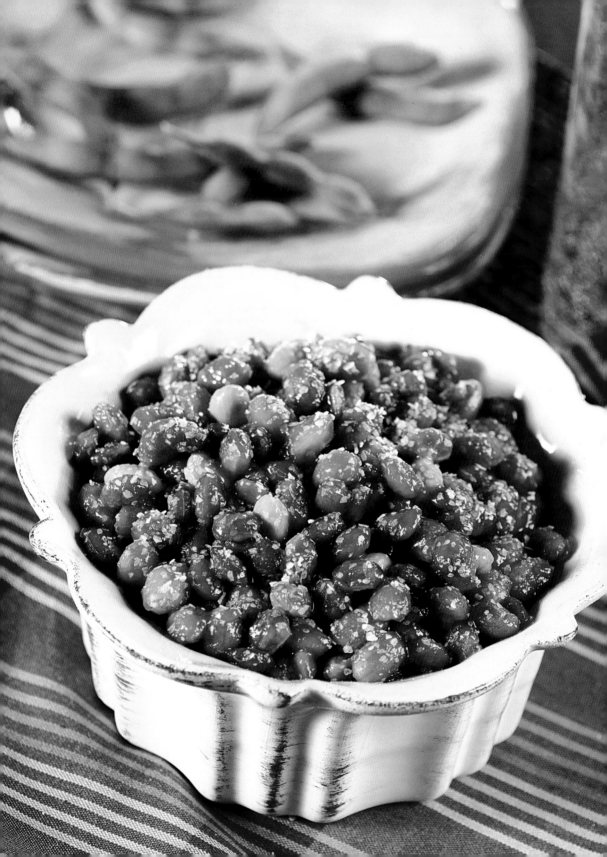

BITE-YOU-BACK
ROASTED EDAMAME

- 2 teaspoons vegetable oil
- 2 teaspoons honey
- ¼ teaspoon wasabi powder
- 1 package (10 ounces) frozen shelled edamame, thawed
- Kosher salt (optional)

1. Preheat oven to 375°F.

2. Combine oil, honey and wasabi powder in large bowl; mix well. Add edamame; toss to coat. Spread on baking sheet in single layer.

3. Bake 12 to 15 minutes or until golden brown, stirring once. Immediately remove from baking sheet to large bowl; sprinkle with salt, if desired. Cool completely before serving. Store in airtight container.

MAKES 4 TO 6 SERVINGS

Calories 78, Total Fat 4g, Saturated Fat 1g, Cholesterol 0mg, Sodium 7mg, Carbohydrates 7g, Dietary Fiber 1g, Protein 4g

KALE CHIPS

1 large bunch kale (about 1 pound)

1 to 2 tablespoons olive oil

1 teaspoon garlic salt or other seasoned salt

1. Preheat oven to 350°F. Line baking sheets with parchment paper.

2. Wash kale and pat dry with paper towels. Remove center ribs and stems; discard. Cut leaves into 2- to 3-inch-wide pieces.

3. Combine leaves, oil and garlic salt in large bowl; toss to coat. Spread on prepared baking sheets.

4. Bake 10 to 15 minutes or until edges are lightly browned and leaves are crisp.* Cool completely on baking sheets. Store in airtight container.

*If the leaves are lightly browned but not crisp, turn oven off and let chips stand in oven until crisp, about 10 minutes. Do not keep the oven on as the chips will burn easily.

MAKES 6 SERVINGS

Calories 43, Total Fat 3g, Saturated Fat 1g, Cholesterol 0mg, Sodium 180mg, Carbohydrates 5g, Dietary Fiber 1g, Protein 2g

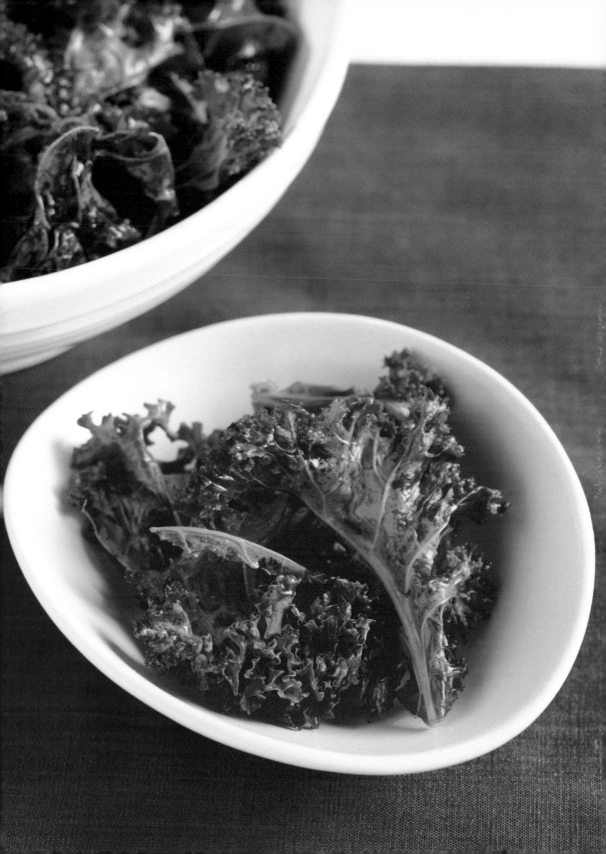

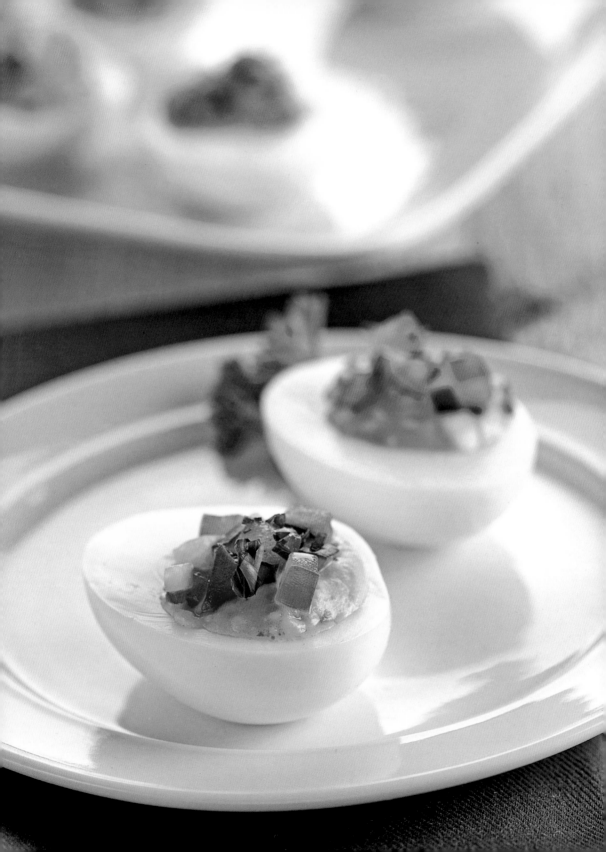

MEDITERRANEAN-STYLE DEVILED EGGS

¼ cup finely diced cucumber

¼ cup finely diced tomato

2 teaspoons fresh lemon juice

⅛ teaspoon salt

6 hard-cooked eggs, peeled and sliced in half lengthwise

⅓ cup roasted garlic or any flavor hummus

Chopped fresh parsley (optional)

1. Combine cucumber, tomato, lemon juice and salt in small bowl; gently mix.

2. Remove yolks from eggs; discard. Spoon 1 heaping teaspoon hummus into each egg half. Top with ½ teaspoon cucumber-tomato mixture and parsley, if desired. Serve immediately.

MAKES 6 SERVINGS

Calories 49, Total Fat 3g, Saturated Fat 0g, Cholesterol 0mg, Sodium 157mg, Carbohydrates 3g, Dietary Fiber 1g, Protein 4g

MINI MARINATED BEEF SKEWERS

1 boneless beef top round steak (about 1 pound)

2 tablespoons reduced-sodium soy sauce

1 tablespoon dry sherry

1 teaspoon dark sesame oil

2 cloves garlic, minced

18 cherry tomatoes (optional)

1. Cut beef crosswise into 18 (⅛-inch) slices. Place in large resealable food storage bag. Combine soy sauce, sherry, sesame oil and garlic in small bowl; pour over beef. Seal bag; turn to coat. Marinate in refrigerator at least 30 minutes or up to 2 hours.

2. Meanwhile, soak 18 (6-inch) wooden skewers in water 20 minutes.

3. Preheat broiler. Drain beef; discard marinade. Weave beef accordion-style onto skewers. Place on rack of broiler pan.

4. Broil 4 to 5 inches from heat 2 minutes. Turn skewers over; broil 2 minutes or until beef is barely pink in center. Garnish with cherry tomatoes; serve warm.

MAKES 18 SERVINGS

Calories 120, Total Fat 4g, Saturated Fat 1g, Cholesterol 60mg, Sodium 99mg, Carbohydrates 2g, Dietary Fiber 1g, Protein 20g

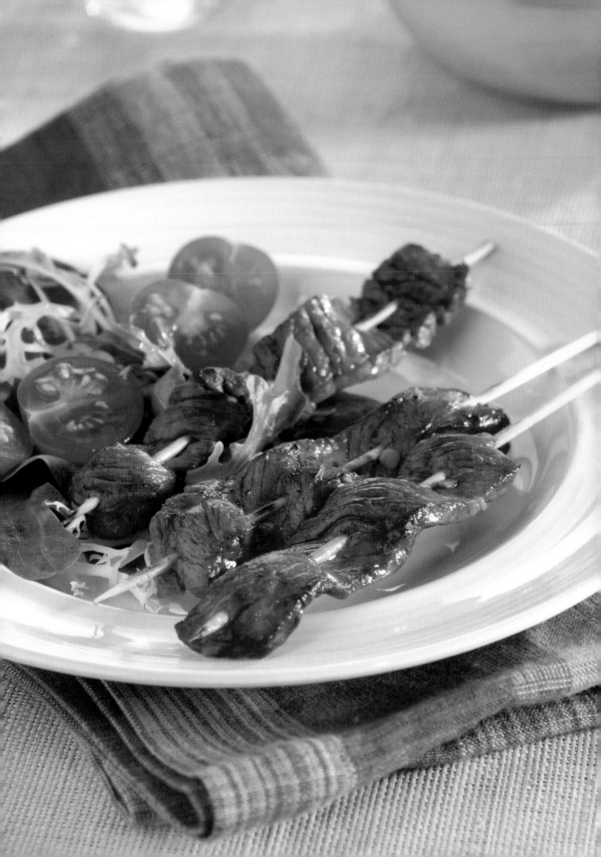

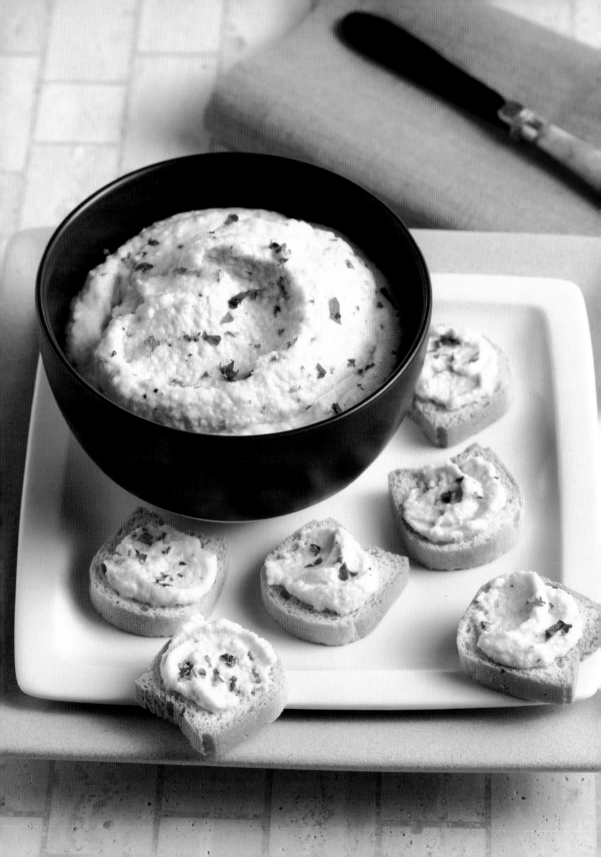

CREAMY CASHEW SPREAD

1 cup raw cashews

2 tablespoons lemon juice

1 tablespoon tahini

½ teaspoon salt

½ teaspoon black pepper

2 teaspoons minced fresh herbs, such as basil, parsley or oregano (optional)

Cut-up vegetables and/or crackers

1. Rinse cashews and place in medium bowl. Cover with water by at least 2 inches. Soak 4 hours or overnight. Drain cashews, reserving soaking water.

2. Place cashews, 2 tablespoons reserved water, lemon juice, tahini, salt and pepper in food processor or blender; process several minutes or until smooth. Add additional water, 1 tablespoon at a time, until desired consistency is reached.

3. Cover and refrigerate until ready to serve. Stir in herbs, if desired, just before serving. Serve with vegetables and/or crackers.

MAKES ABOUT ½ CUP (6 SERVINGS)

Tip: *Use as a spread or dip for hors d'oeuvres, or as a sandwich spread or pasta topping. Thin with additional liquid as needed.*

Calories 136, Total Fat 11g, Saturated Fat 2g, Cholesterol 0mg, Sodium 197mg, Carbohydrates 8g, Dietary Fiber 1g, Protein 4g

EGG WHITE SALAD CUCUMBER BOATS

6 hard-cooked eggs, peeled

⅓ cup light mayonnaise

Juice of 1 lemon

1 teaspoon fresh dill, plus additional for garnish

¼ teaspoon salt

¼ cup finely chopped green bell pepper

¼ cup finely chopped red bell pepper

2 tablespoons finely chopped red onion

1 English cucumber

1. Slice eggs in half lengthwise; discard yolks. Finely grate or chop egg whites.

2. Whisk mayonnaise, lemon juice, 1 teaspoon dill and salt in medium bowl. Gently stir in egg whites, bell peppers and onion.

3. Cut cucumber in half crosswise; cut each piece in half lengthwise to make 4 equal pieces. Scoop out cucumber pieces with rounded ½ teaspoon, leaving thick shell.

4. Fill each shell evenly with egg white salad. Garnish with additional dill.

MAKES 2 SERVINGS

Calories 175, Total Fat 9g, Saturated Fat 1g, Cholesterol 6mg, Sodium 756mg, Carbohydrates 11g, Dietary Fiber 1g, Protein 12g

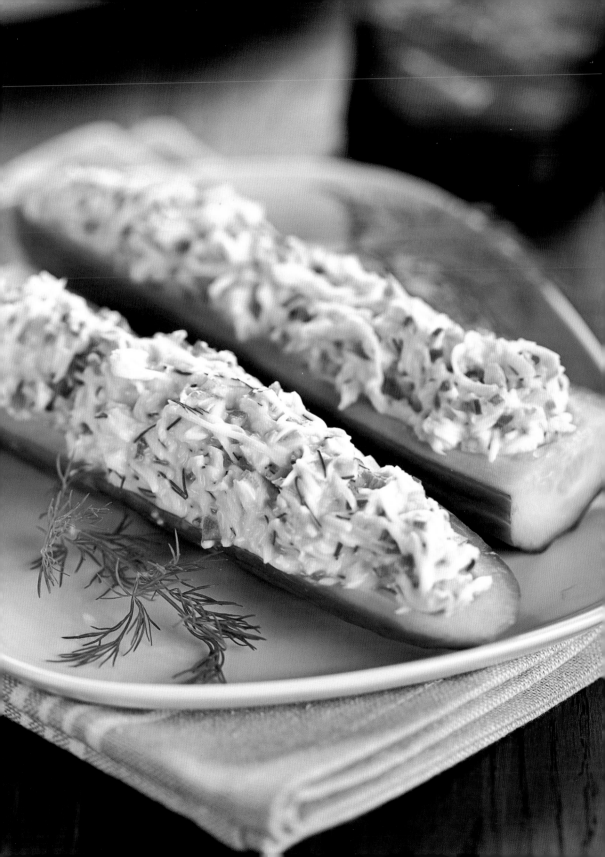

SALADS

CHICKEN AND APPLE SPRING GREENS WITH POPPY SEEDS

1 package (5 ounces) spring salad greens

12 ounces cooked chicken strips

1 large Golden Delicious apple, thinly sliced

⅓ cup thinly sliced red onion

1 ounce crumbled goat cheese (optional)

¼ cup cider vinegar

2 tablespoons canola oil

½ teaspoon poppy seeds

¼ teaspoon salt

⅛ teaspoon red pepper flakes

1. Arrange greens, chicken, apple and onion on evenly on four plates. Sprinkle with cheese, if desired.

2. Combine vinegar, oil, poppy seeds, salt and red pepper flakes in small jar with tight-fitting lid; shake well. Drizzle dressing over salads.

MAKES 4 SERVINGS

Calories 224, Total Fat 10g, Saturated Fat 1g, Cholesterol 43mg, Sodium 206mg, Carbohydrates 8g, Dietary Fiber 2g, Protein 26g

SUMMER SZECHUAN TOFU SALAD

¼ cup reduced-sodium soy sauce

1 tablespoon canola or peanut oil

1 tablespoon dark sesame oil

1 teaspoon minced fresh ginger

½ teaspoon hot pepper sauce

1 package extra-firm tofu

4 cups baby spinach leaves

4 cups sliced napa cabbage or romaine lettuce leaves

2 cups diagonally halved fresh sugar snap peas or snow peas

1 cup julienned carrots

1 cup fresh bean sprouts

¼ cup dry-roasted peanuts or toasted slivered almonds

Chopped fresh cilantro or green onions (optional)

1. Whisk soy sauce, canola oil, sesame oil, ginger and hot pepper sauce in small bowl.

2. Drain tofu and place between layers of paper towels. Press lightly to drain excess water from tofu. Cut tofu into 1-inch cubes. Place in shallow dish. Drizzle 2 tablespoons soy sauce mixture over tofu cubes. Set aside.

3. Combine spinach, cabbage, sugar snap peas, carrots and bean sprouts in large bowl. Add remaining soy sauce mixture. Toss well. Transfer to plates. Top with tofu mixture, peanuts and cilantro, if desired.

MAKES 4 SERVINGS

Calories 223, Total Fat 12g, Saturated Fat 2g, Cholesterol 0mg, Sodium 655mg, Carbohydrates 18g, Dietary Fiber 5g, Protein 14g

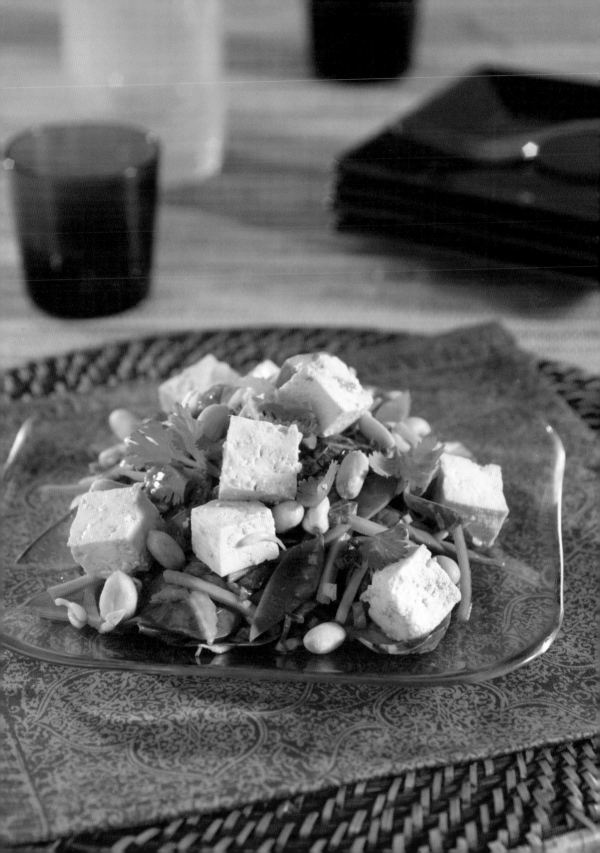

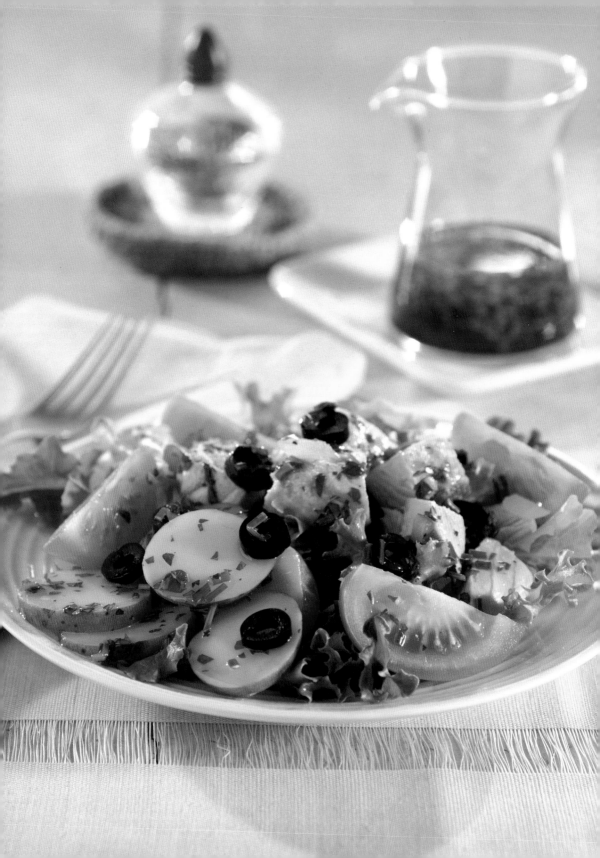

WARM SALMON SALAD

Chive Vinaigrette
(recipe follows)

2 cups water

¼ cup chopped
onion

2 tablespoons red
wine vinegar

¼ teaspoon black
pepper

1¼ pounds small
unpeeled red
potatoes

1 pound salmon
steaks

6 cups torn washed
mixed salad
greens

2 medium
tomatoes, cut
into wedges

16 kalamata olives,
sliced

1. Prepare Chive Vinaigrette.

2. Combine water, onion, vinegar and pepper in large saucepan; bring to a boil over medium-high heat. Add potatoes. Cover; simmer 10 minutes or until fork-tender. Transfer potatoes to cutting board using slotted spoon; cool slightly. Reserve water.

3. Cut potatoes into thick slices; place in medium bowl. Toss potatoes with ⅓ cup Chive Vinaigrette; set aside.

4. Rinse salmon and pat dry with paper towels. Add fish to reserved water and simmer gently 4 to 5 minutes or until fish is opaque and flakes easily when tested with fork. *Do not boil.*

5. Carefully remove fish from water with slotted spatula; place on cutting board. Let stand 5 minutes. Remove skin and bones from fish; cut into 1-inch cubes.

6. Place salad greens onto four plates. Top with fish, potatoes, tomatoes and olives. Drizzle with remaining Chive Vinaigrette.

MAKES 4 SERVINGS

CHIVE VINAIGRETTE

⅓ cup vegetable oil

¼ cup red wine vinegar

2 tablespoons finely chopped
fresh chives

2 tablespoons finely chopped
fresh parsley

⅛ teaspoon salt

⅛ teaspoon white pepper

Combine oil, vinegar, chives, parsley, salt and pepper in jar with tight-fitting lid; shake well to combine. Refrigerate until ready to use.

Calories 610, **Total Fat** 42g, **Saturated Fat** 6g, **Cholesterol** 60mg, **Sodium** 670mg, **Carbohydrates** 32g, **Dietary Fiber** 5g, **Protein** 28g

GREEK LENTIL SALAD WITH FETA VINAIGRETTE

4 cups water

¾ cup uncooked lentils

1 bay leaf

1 cup grape tomatoes, halved

1 stalk celery, chopped

¼ cup chopped green onions

¼ cup crumbled feta cheese

2 tablespoons olive oil

1 tablespoon white wine vinegar

½ teaspoon dried thyme

½ teaspoon dried oregano

½ teaspoon salt

¼ teaspoon black pepper

1. Combine water, lentils and bay leaf in small saucepan. Bring to a boil. Reduce heat to medium-low; partially cover and cook 40 minutes or until lentils are tender but not mushy.

2. Drain lentils; remove and discard bay leaf. Place lentils in serving bowl; stir in tomatoes, celery and green onions.

3. Combine feta, oil, vinegar, thyme, oregano, salt and pepper in small bowl. Pour over salad; gently stir until blended. Let stand at least 10 minutes before serving to allow flavors to blend.

MAKES 3 SERVINGS

Calories 310, Total Fat 13g, Saturated Fat 3g, Cholesterol 5mg, Sodium 530mg, Carbohydrates 36g, Dietary Fiber 16g, Protein 16g

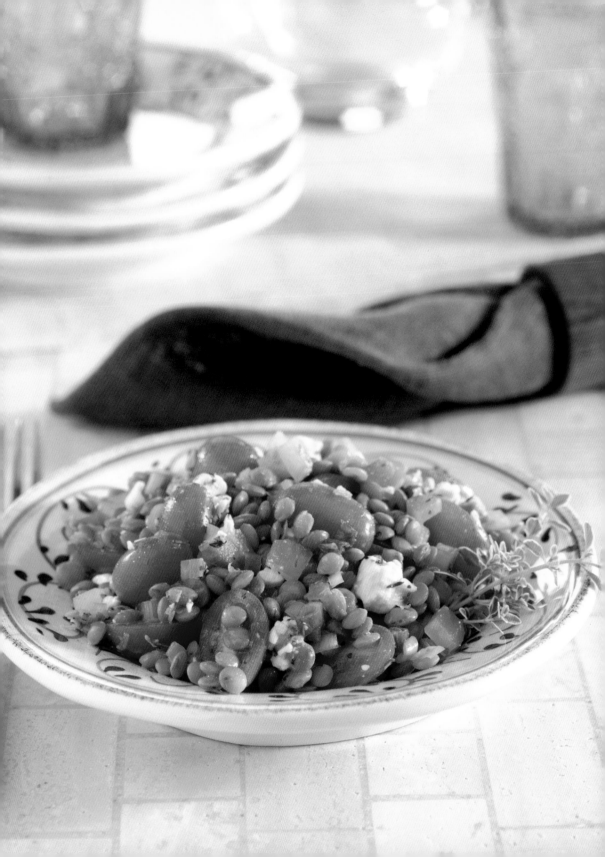

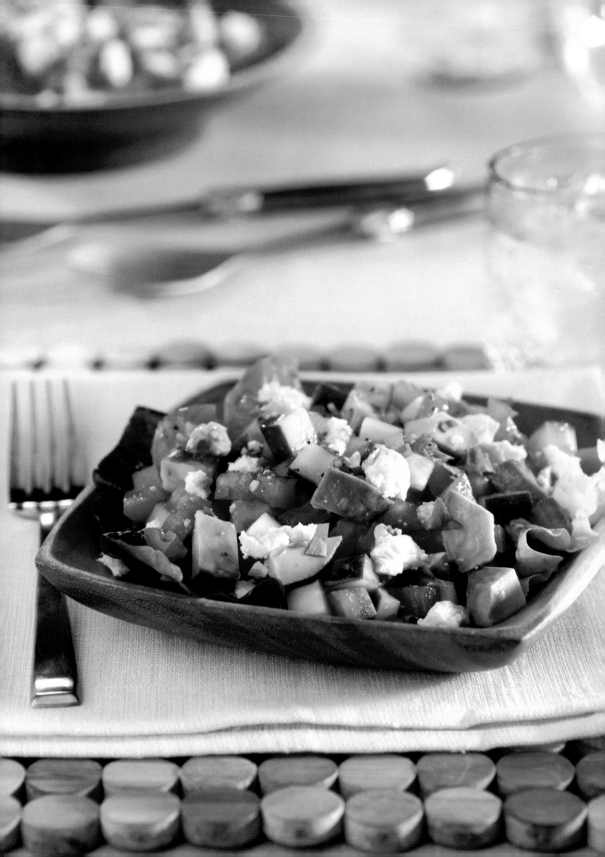

TOMATO, AVOCADO AND CUCUMBER SALAD

1½ tablespoons extra virgin olive oil

1 tablespoon balsamic vinegar

1 clove garlic, minced

¼ teaspoon salt

¼ teaspoon black pepper

2 cups diced seeded plum tomatoes

1 small ripe avocado, diced into ½-inch chunks

½ cup chopped cucumber

⅓ cup crumbled reduced-fat feta cheese

4 large red leaf lettuce leaves

Chopped fresh basil (optional)

1. Whisk oil, vinegar, garlic, salt and pepper in medium bowl. Add tomatoes and avocado; toss to coat evenly. Gently stir in cucumber and feta cheese.

2. Arrange lettuce on four serving plates. Spoon salad evenly onto lettuce leaves; top with basil, if desired.

MAKES 4 SERVINGS

Calories 138, Total Fat 11g, Saturated Fat 2g, Cholesterol 3mg, Sodium 311mg, Carbohydrates 7g, Dietary Fiber 2g, Protein 4g

FLANK STEAK AND ROASTED VEGETABLE SALAD

1½ pounds asparagus spears, trimmed and cut into 2-inch lengths

1¾ cups baby carrots (8 ounces)

1 tablespoon plus 1 teaspoon olive oil, divided

¾ teaspoon salt, divided

1 teaspoon black pepper, divided

1 pound flank steak (1 inch thick)

2 tablespoons plus 1 teaspoon Dijon mustard, divided

1 tablespoon fresh lemon juice

1 tablespoon water

1 teaspoon honey

6 cups mixed salad greens

1. Preheat oven to 400°F. Place asparagus and carrots in shallow roasting pan. Drizzle with 1 teaspoon oil; sprinkle with ¼ teaspoon salt and ¼ teaspoon pepper. Toss to coat. Bake 20 minutes, stirring once, until vegetables are browned and tender.

2. Meanwhile, sprinkle steak with ¼ teaspoon salt and ½ teaspoon pepper. Rub both sides of steak with 2 tablespoons mustard. Place steak on rack in baking pan. Bake 10 minutes for medium-rare or to desired doneness, turning once. Let stand 5 minutes; cut across the grain into thin slices.

3. Whisk lemon juice, remaining 1 tablespoon oil, water, honey, remaining 1 teaspoon mustard, ¼ teaspoon salt and ¼ teaspoon pepper in large bowl.

4. Drizzle 1 tablespoon dressing over vegetables in pan; toss to coat. Add greens to remaining dressing; toss to coat. Divide greens among serving plates. Top with steak and vegetables.

MAKES 4 SERVINGS

Calories 300, Total Fat 13g, Saturated Fat 4g, Cholesterol 46mg, Sodium 747mg, Carbohydrates 16g, Dietary Fiber 6g, Protein 32g

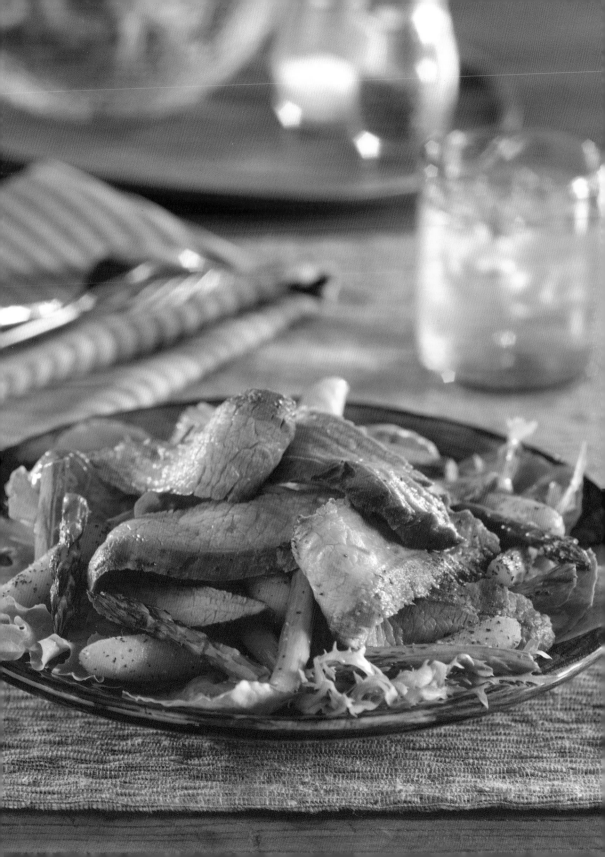

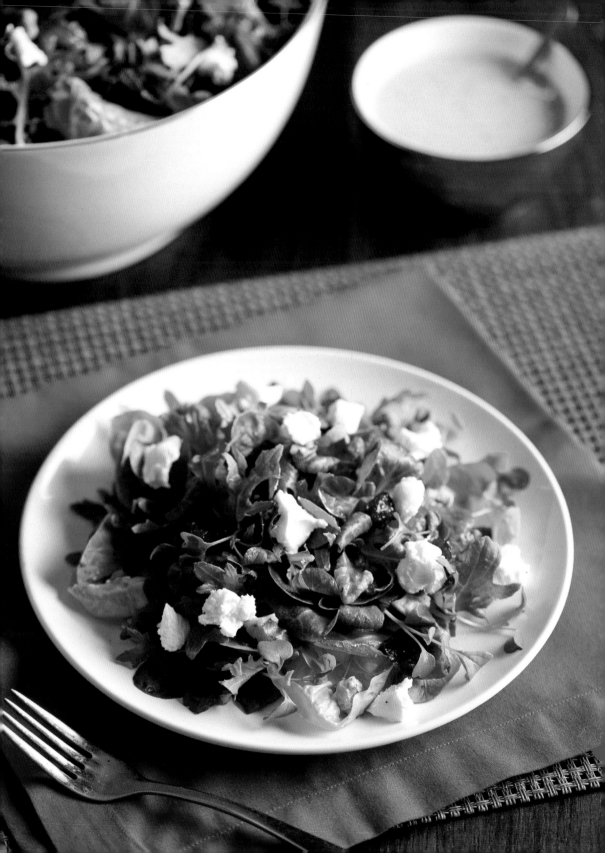

MESCLUN SALAD WITH CRANBERRY VINAIGRETTE

DRESSING

- ⅓ **cup extra virgin olive oil**
- 3 **tablespoons champagne vinegar or sherry vinegar**
- 1 **tablespoon Dijon mustard**
- ¾ **teaspoon salt**
- ¼ **teaspoon black pepper**

SALAD

- 10 **cups (10 ounces) mesclun or mixed torn salad greens**
- 4 **ounces goat cheese, crumbled**
- ½ **cup dried cranberries**
- ½ **cup walnuts or pecans, coarsely chopped and toasted***

*To toast nuts, spread in single layer on baking sheet. Bake in preheated 350°F oven 8 to 10 minutes or until golden brown, stirring frequently.

1. For dressing, whisk oil, vinegar, mustard, salt and pepper in small bowl. Cover and refrigerate at least 30 minutes or up to 24 hours before serving.

2. For salad, combine greens, goat cheese, cranberries and walnuts in large bowl. Whisk dressing again and add to salad; toss until evenly coated.

MAKES 8 SERVINGS

Calories 233, **Total Fat** 19g, **Saturated Fat** 5g, **Cholesterol** 15mg, **Sodium** 325mg, **Carbohydrates** 10g, **Dietary Fiber** 2.5g, **Protein** 7g

MANGO CRAB SALAD

1 mango

2 tablespoons fresh lime juice

2 tablespoons olive oil

½ teaspoon salt

¼ teaspoon ground ginger

¼ teaspoon ground red pepper

8 ounces lump crabmeat*

1 package (10 ounces) mixed salad greens

2 green onions, thinly sliced

1 avocado, thinly sliced

½ cup chopped fresh cilantro

Pick out and discard any pieces of shell or cartilage.

1. Finely dice mango to equal ¼ cup; set remaining mango aside. Place finely diced mango in large bowl; stir in lime juice, oil, salt, ginger and red pepper until well blended. Transfer 2 tablespoons dressing to another large bowl. Add crabmeat to dressing in first bowl.

2. Cut remaining mango into ½-inch cubes. Add mango, salad greens and green onions to remaining dressing; toss to blend. Divide evenly among four salad plates; top with crabmeat mixture, avocado and cilantro.

MAKES 4 SERVINGS

Calories 260, **Total Fat** 15g, **Saturated Fat** 3g, **Cholesterol** 55mg, **Sodium** 540mg, **Carbohydrates** 22g, **Dietary Fiber** 7g, **Protein** 13g

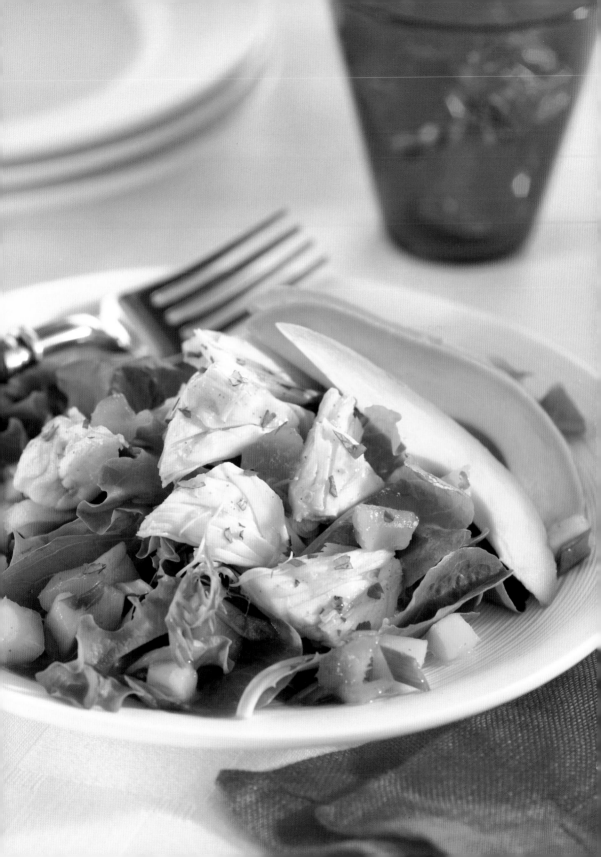

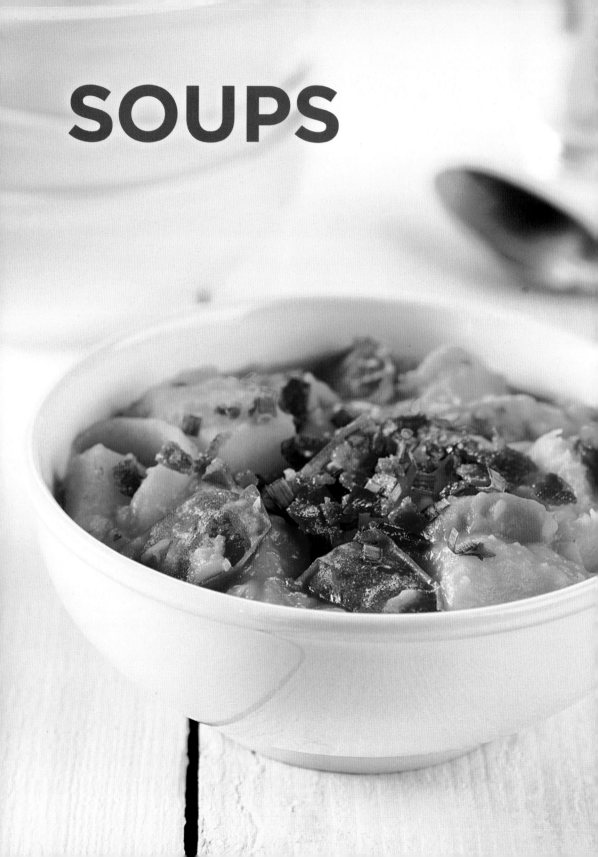

SOUPS

HEARTY LENTIL AND ROOT VEGETABLE STEW

2 cans (about 14 ounces each) chicken or vegetable broth

1½ cups diced turnip

1 cup dried red lentils, rinsed and sorted

1 medium onion, cut into ½-inch wedges

2 medium carrots, cut into 1-inch pieces

1 medium red bell pepper, cut into 1-inch pieces

½ teaspoon dried oregano

⅛ teaspoon red pepper flakes

1 tablespoon olive oil

½ teaspoon salt

4 slices bacon, crisp-cooked and crumbled (optional)

½ cup finely chopped green onions

SLOW COOKER DIRECTIONS

1. Combine broth, turnip, lentils, onion, carrots, bell pepper, oregano and red pepper flakes in 4-quart slow cooker. Cover; cook on LOW 6 hours or on HIGH 3 hours or until lentils are tender.

2. Stir in oil and salt. Sprinkle each serving with bacon, if desired, and green onions.

MAKES 8 SERVINGS

Calories 164, **Total Fat** 4g, **Saturated Fat** 1g, **Cholesterol** 14mg, **Sodium** 355mg, **Carbohydrates** 21g, **Dietary Fiber** 9g, **Protein** 12g

SALMON AND WILD RICE CHOWDER

1   teaspoon olive oil

1   red onion, chopped

1   red bell pepper, chopped

1   cup fresh or frozen green beans, cut into 1-inch pieces

1½ teaspoons minced fresh dill weed

1   teaspoon salt

⅛   teaspoon black pepper

3   cups vegetable broth

1   cup cooked wild rice

12 ounces skinless salmon fillet, cut into 1-inch pieces

2   teaspoons all-purpose flour

½   cup milk

1. Heat oil in large saucepan over high heat. Add onion, bell pepper and green beans; cook and stir 5 minutes. Stir in dill, salt and black pepper. Pour in broth; bring to a simmer.

2. Add wild rice and salmon to saucepan. Reduce heat to low; cover and simmer 6 to 8 minutes or until salmon flakes easily when tested with fork.

3. Place flour in small bowl. Slowly whisk in milk. Stir into saucepan. Cook until heated through.

MAKES 8 SERVINGS

Calories 115, Total Fat 4g, Saturated Fat 1g, Cholesterol 24mg, Sodium 441mg, Carbohydrates 11g, Dietary Fiber 1g, Protein 11g

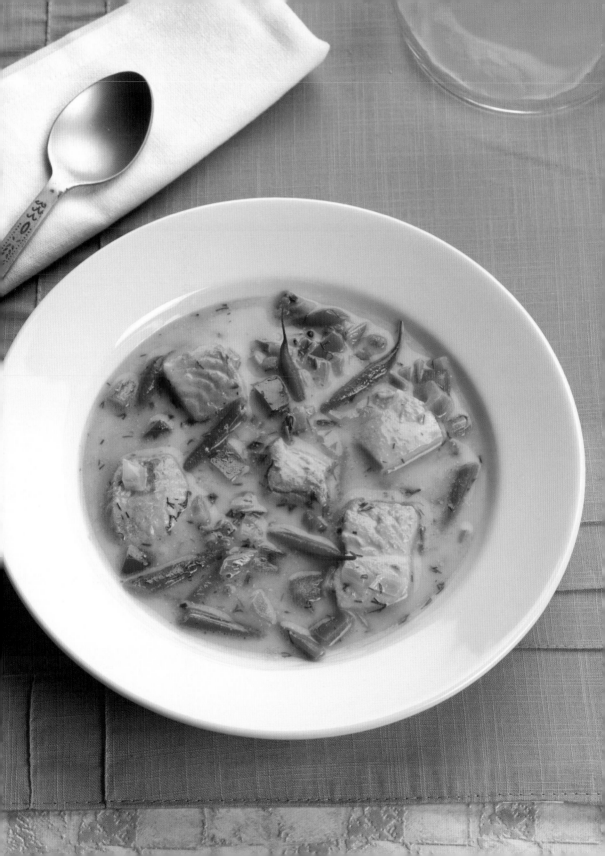

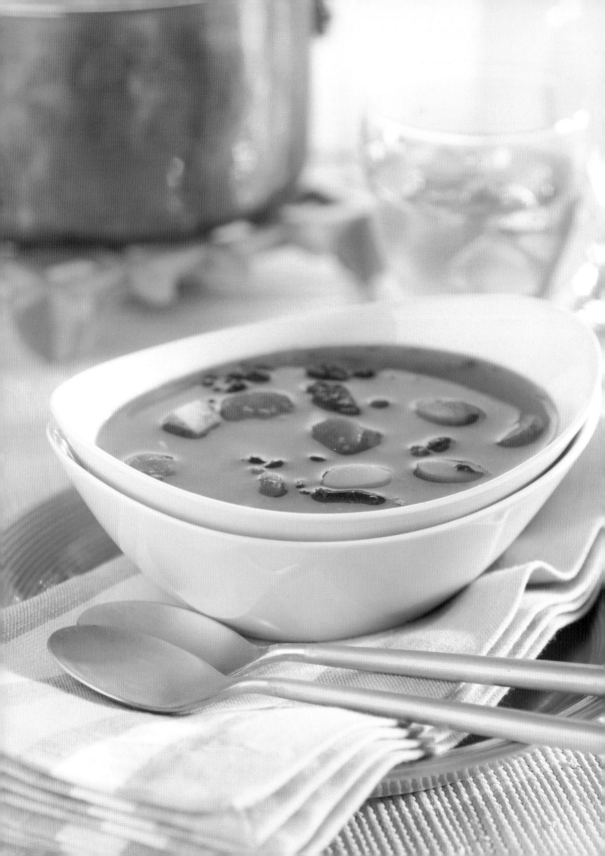

KALE AND WHITE BEAN SOUP

2 slices reduced-sodium bacon, chopped

½ cup diced onion

1 unpeeled new red potato, diced

2 cans (about 14 ounces each) reduced-sodium vegetable broth

1 teaspoon minced garlic

½ teaspoon dried oregano

2 bay leaves

1 can (14½ ounces) low-sodium sliced carrots, drained

1 can (13½ ounces) kale or spinach, drained

1 can (10 ounces) reduced-sodium white kidney beans, rinsed and drained

⅓ cup finely chopped oil-packed sun-dried tomato strips

1 tablespoon olive oil

¼ teaspoon black pepper

⅛ teaspoon salt

1. Cook bacon in large saucepan over medium heat until crisp. Drain fat.

2. Add onion and potato to saucepan; cook and stir 10 minutes or until onion is browned. Stir in broth, garlic, oregano and bay leaves; bring to a simmer. Cover and simmer 5 minutes or until potato is tender.

3. Add carrots, kale, beans and sun-dried tomatoes; cook 5 minutes. Remove and discard bay leaves. Stir in oil, pepper and salt.

MAKES 6 SERVINGS

Calories 165, Total Fat 5g, Saturated Fat 1g, Cholesterol 2mg, Sodium 479mg, Carbohydrates 24g, Dietary Fiber 6g, Protein 7g

CHUNKY CHICKEN STEW

1 teaspoon olive oil

1 small onion, chopped

1 cup thinly sliced carrots

1 cup reduced-sodium chicken broth

1 can (about 14 ounces) diced tomatoes

1 cup diced cooked chicken breast

3 cups sliced kale or baby spinach

1. Heat oil in large saucepan over medium-high heat. Add onion; cook and stir about 5 minutes or until golden brown. Stir in carrots and broth; bring to a boil. Reduce heat; simmer, uncovered, 5 minutes.

2. Stir in tomatoes; simmer 5 minutes or until carrots are tender. Add chicken; cook and stir until heated through. Add kale; stir until wilted.

MAKES 2 SERVINGS

Calories 287, Total Fat 6g, Saturated Fat 1g, Cholesterol 66mg, Sodium 337mg, Carbohydrates 30g, Dietary Fiber 8g, Protein 30g

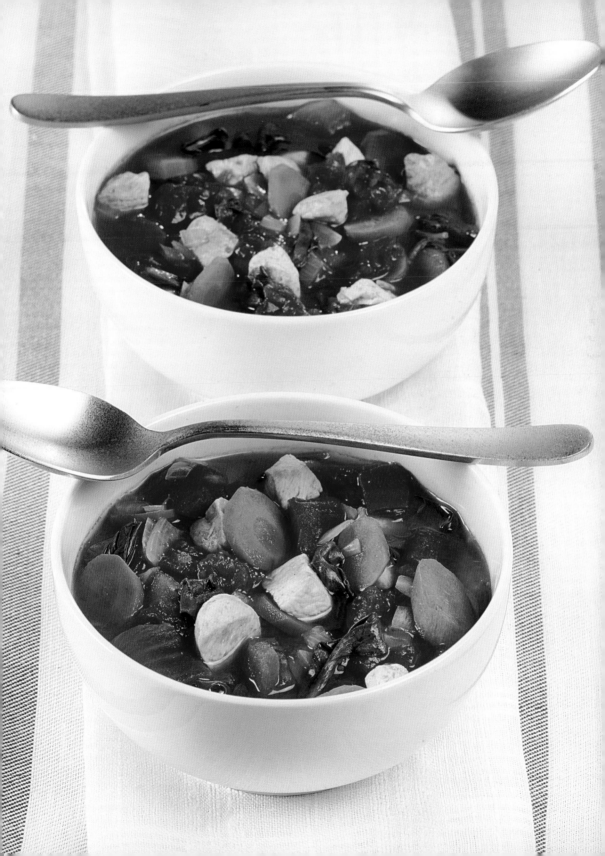

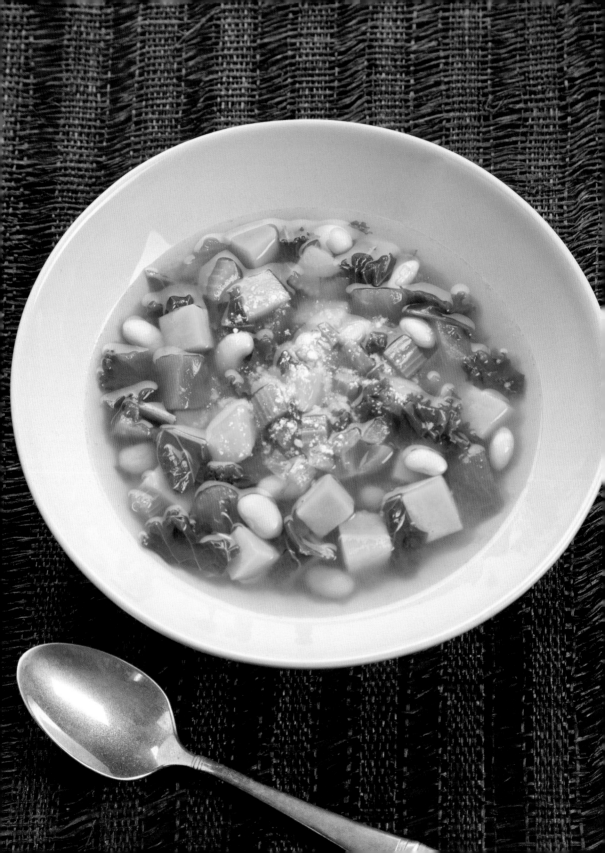

SWEET POTATO MINESTRONE

- 1 tablespoon extra virgin olive oil
- ¾ cup diced onion
- ½ cup diced celery
- 3 cups water
- 2 cups diced peeled sweet potatoes
- 1 can (about 15 ounces) Great Northern beans, rinsed and drained
- 1 can (about 14 ounces) no-salt-added diced tomatoes
- ¾ teaspoon dried rosemary
- ½ teaspoon salt (optional)
- ⅛ teaspoon black pepper
- 2 cups coarsely chopped kale leaves (lightly packed)
- 4 tablespoons grated Parmesan cheese

1. Heat oil in large saucepan or Dutch oven over medium-high heat. Add onion and celery; cook and stir 4 minutes or until onion is softened. Stir water, sweet potatoes, beans, tomatoes, rosemary, salt, if desired, and pepper into saucepan. Cover and bring to a simmer; reduce heat and simmer 30 minutes.

2. Add kale; cover and cook 10 minutes or until tender.

3. Ladle soup into bowls; sprinkle with cheese.

MAKES 4 SERVINGS

Note: *Choose kale in small bunches with firm leaves and a rich, deep color. Avoid bunches with limp, wilted or discolored leaves. To remove the tough stems, make a "V-shaped" cut where the stem joins the leaf. Stack the leaves and cut them into pieces.*

Calories 286, Total Fat 6g, Saturated Fat 2g, Cholesterol 4mg, Sodium 189mg, Carbohydrates 48g, Dietary Fiber 11g, Protein 13g

TURKEY ALBONDIGAS SOUP

¼ cup uncooked brown rice

MEATBALLS

8 ounces ground turkey

1 tablespoon minced onion

1 teaspoon chopped fresh cilantro

1 teaspoon milk

½ teaspoon hot pepper sauce

⅛ teaspoon dried oregano

⅛ teaspoon black pepper

BROTH

1 teaspoon olive oil

2 tablespoons chopped onion

1 clove garlic, minced

2½ cups reduced-sodium chicken broth

2 teaspoons hot pepper sauce

1 teaspoon tomato paste

⅛ teaspoon black pepper

3 carrots, sliced (about 1 cup)

½ zucchini, quartered lengthwise and cut crosswise into ½-inch slices

½ yellow squash, quartered lengthwise and sliced

Lime wedges and chopped fresh cilantro (optional)

1. Prepare rice according to package directions.

2. Meanwhile, combine turkey, 1 tablespoon minced onion, 1 teaspoon chopped cilantro, milk, ½ teaspoon hot pepper sauce, oregano and ⅛ teaspoon black pepper in medium bowl. Mix lightly until blended. Shape mixture into 1-inch balls.

3. For broth, heat oil in large saucepan over medium heat. Add 2 tablespoons onion and garlic; cook and stir until golden. Add broth, 2 teaspoons hot pepper sauce, tomato paste and ⅛ teaspoon black pepper. Bring to a boil over high heat; reduce to simmer.

4. Add meatballs and carrots to broth; simmer 15 minutes. Add zucchini, squash and cooked rice. Simmer 5 to 10 minutes or just until vegetables are tender. Ladle into bowls. Serve immediately with lime wedges and cilantro, if desired.

MAKES 2 SERVINGS

Calories 342, Total Fat 11g, Saturated Fat 3g, Cholesterol 70mg, Sodium 404mg, Carbohydrates 32g, Dietary Fiber 5g, Protein 30g

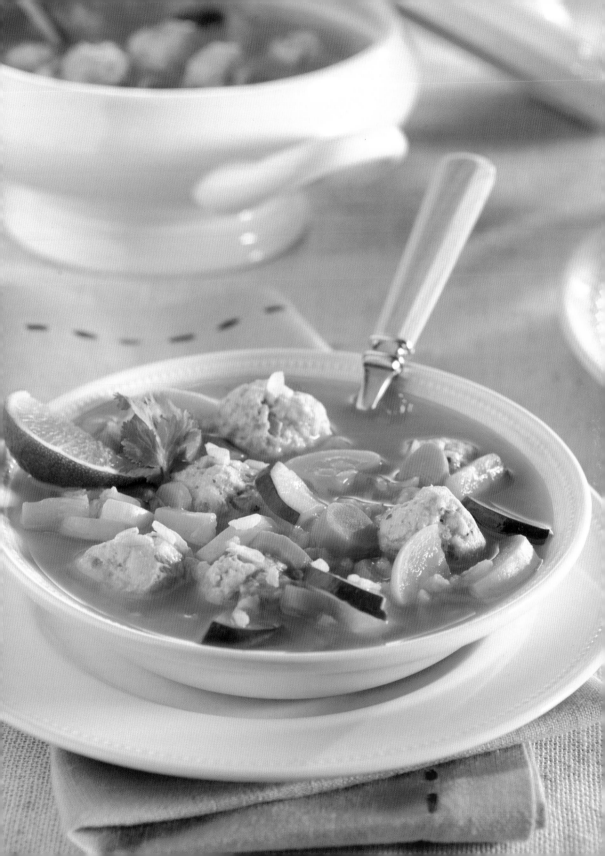

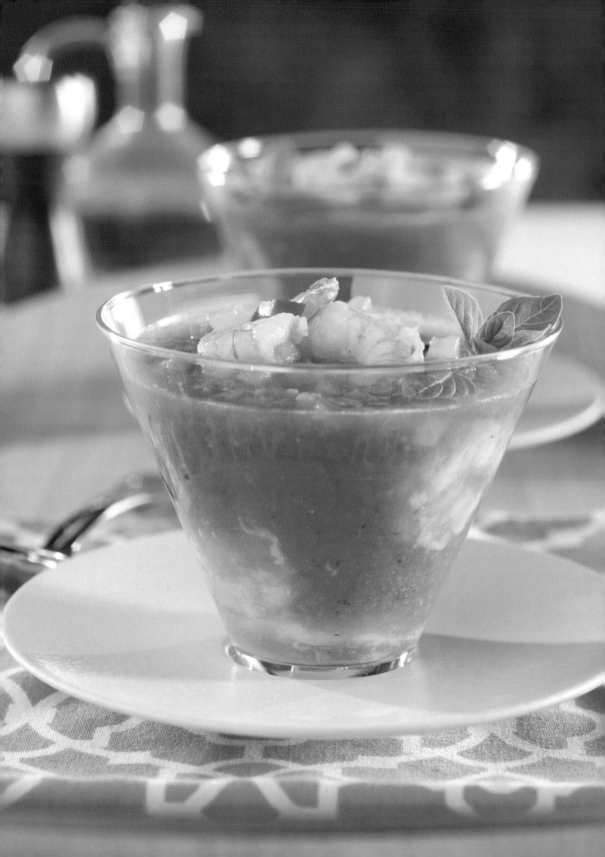

SHRIMP GAZPACHO

1 teaspoon olive oil

8 ounces medium raw shrimp, peeled and deveined, tails removed

⅛ teaspoon salt (optional)

⅛ teaspoon black pepper

3 plum tomatoes, chopped (about 1½ cups)

¼ small red onion, chopped

1 clove garlic, chopped

¼ cucumber, peeled and chopped

¼ cup finely chopped jarred roasted bell peppers (red and/or yellow), divided

¾ cup tomato juice

1 tablespoon red wine vinegar

1. Heat oil in medium nonstick skillet over high heat, swirling to coat. Season shrimp with salt, if desired, and black pepper. Cook 3 minutes or until browned on both sides and opaque in center; transfer to plate.

2. Combine tomatoes, onion, garlic, cucumber and half roasted peppers in food processor; process until combined. Add tomato juice and vinegar; process until smooth.

3. Divide soup among bowls; top with shrimp and remaining roasted peppers.

MAKES 2 SERVINGS

Calories 202, Total Fat 5g, Saturated Fat 1g, Cholesterol 172mg, Sodium 464mg, Carbohydrates 16g, Dietary Fiber 2g, Protein 25g

CURRIED VEGETABLE AND CASHEW STEW

2 medium potatoes, peeled and cut into ½-inch cubes

12 ounces eggplant, cut into ½-inch cubes

1 can (about 15 ounces) chickpeas, rinsed and drained

1 medium onion, chopped

1 can (about 14 ounces) petite diced tomatoes

1 cup vegetable broth

2 tablespoons quick cooking tapioca

2 teaspoons grated fresh ginger

2 teaspoons curry powder

½ teaspoon salt

¼ teaspoon black pepper

1 medium zucchini (about 8 ounces), cut into ½-inch cubes

1 cup golden raisins

½ cup frozen peas

½ cup lightly salted cashews

SLOW COOKER DIRECTIONS

1. Combine potatoes, eggplant, chickpeas, onion, tomatoes, broth, tapioca, ginger, curry powder, salt and pepper in slow cooker. Cover; cook on LOW 8 to 9 hours.

2. Stir zucchini, raisins, peas and cashews into slow cooker. *Turn slow cooker to HIGH.* Cover; cook 1 hour or until zucchini is tender.

MAKES 6 SERVINGS

Calories 210, **Total Fat** 70g, **Saturated Fat** 2g, **Cholesterol** 0mg, **Sodium** 230mg, **Carbohydrates** 28g, **Dietary Fiber** 6g, **Protein** 8g

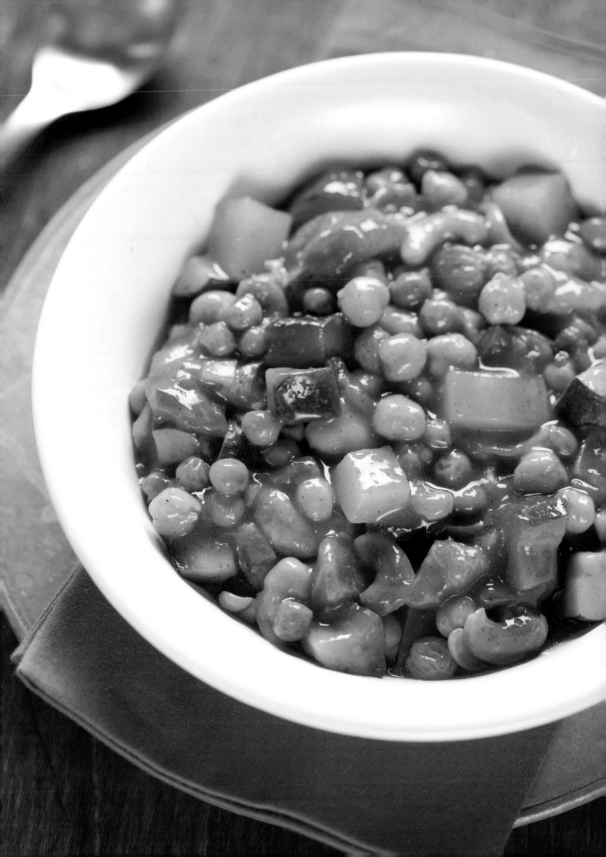

MEAT & CHICKEN

ITALIAN–STYLE POT ROAST

- 2 teaspoons minced garlic
- 1 teaspoon salt
- 1 teaspoon dried basil
- 1 teaspoon dried oregano
- ¼ teaspoon red pepper flakes
- 1 boneless beef bottom round or chuck roast (2½ to 3 pounds)
- 1 onion, quartered and thinly sliced
- 1 can (about 14 ounces) crushed tomatoes
- 2 cans (about 15 ounces each) cannellini or Great Northern beans, rinsed and drained
- ¼ cup thinly sliced fresh basil or chopped Italian parsley

SLOW COOKER DIRECTIONS

1. Combine garlic, salt, dried basil, oregano and red pepper flakes in small bowl; rub over roast.

2. Place half of onion slices in slow cooker. Cut roast in half crosswise. Place half of roast over onion slices; top with remaining onion slices and other half of roast. Pour tomatoes over roast. Cover; cook on LOW 8 to 9 hours or until roast is fork-tender.

3. Remove roast to cutting board; tent with foil. Let liquid in slow cooker stand 5 minutes. Skim off fat.

4. *Turn slow cooker to HIGH.* Stir beans into liquid. Cover; cook 15 to 30 minutes or until beans are heated through. Carve roast across grain into thin slices. Serve with bean mixture and fresh basil.

MAKES 8 SERVINGS

Calories 300, **Total Fat** 6g, **Saturated Fat** 2g, Cholesterol 85mg, **Sodium** 750mg, **Carbohydrates** 22g, Dietary Fiber 7g, Protein 39g

FORTY-CLOVE CHICKEN FILICE

¼ cup olive oil

1 whole chicken (about 3 pounds), cut into pieces

40 cloves garlic (about 2 heads), peeled

4 stalks celery, thickly sliced

½ cup chicken broth

¼ cup dry vermouth

Grated peel and juice of 1 lemon

2 tablespoons finely chopped fresh parsley

2 teaspoons dried basil

1 teaspoon dried oregano

Pinch of red pepper flakes

Salt and black pepper

1. Preheat oven to 375°F.

2. Heat oil in Dutch oven. Add chicken; cook until browned on all sides.

3. Combine garlic, celery, broth, vermouth, lemon peel and juice, parsley, basil, oregano and red pepper flakes in medium bowl; pour over chicken. Season with salt and black pepper.

4. Cover and bake 40 minutes. Remove cover; bake 15 minutes or until chicken is cooked through (165°F).

MAKES 4 TO 6 SERVINGS

Calories 400, Total Fat 22g, Saturated Fat 5g, Cholesterol 100mg, Sodium 240mg, Carbohydrates 13g, Dietary Fiber 2g, Protein 34g

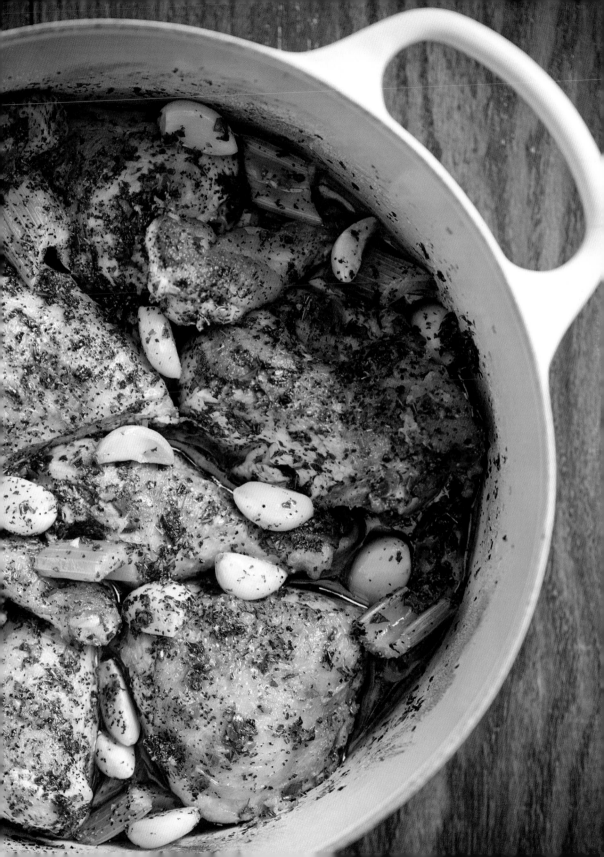

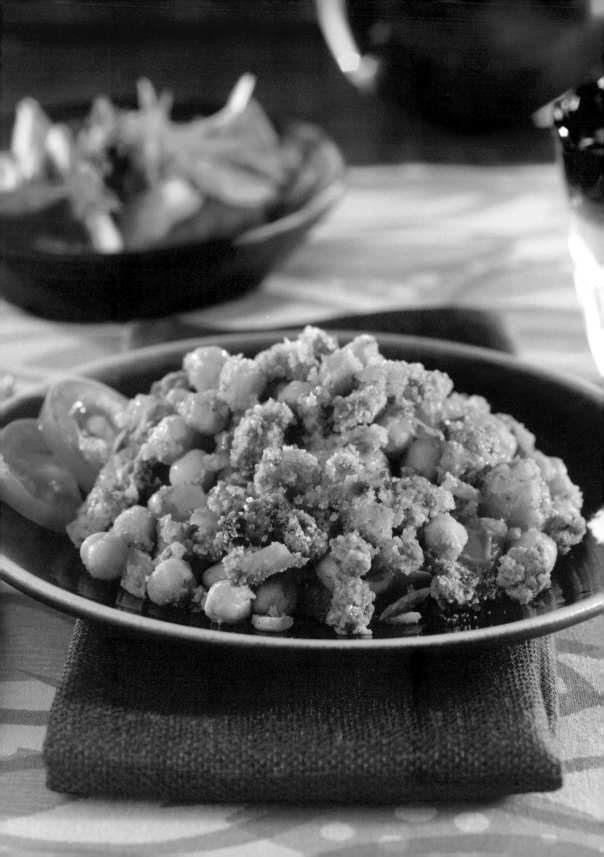

INDIAN–STYLE LAMB AND CHICKPEAS

2 tablespoons butter, divided

1 onion, chopped

3 cloves garlic, chopped

2 teaspoons finely chopped fresh ginger

1 pound ground lamb

Salt and black pepper

1 pound fresh tomatoes (about 3 medium), diced

1 tablespoon curry powder

½ teaspoon ground red pepper

⅛ teaspoon ground cinnamon

⅛ teaspoon ground nutmeg

2 cans (about 15 ounces each) chickpeas, rinsed and drained

¾ cup plain yogurt (not non-fat)

½ cup finely chopped cashews (optional)

¼ cup plain dry bread crumbs (optional)

1. Preheat oven to 350°F.

2. Melt 1 tablespoon butter in large skillet over medium-high heat. Add onion, garlic and ginger; cook and stir 2 minutes or until onion begins to soften. Add lamb; cook until no longer pink, stirring to break up meat. Season with salt and black pepper.

3. Add tomatoes, curry powder, red pepper, cinnamon and nutmeg; cook and stir 5 minutes. Remove from heat. Add chickpeas and yogurt; stir to combine. Transfer mixture to 2- to 2½-quart casserole.

4. Bake 20 minutes. Sprinkle with cashews and bread crumbs, if desired, and dot with remaining 1 tablespoon butter. Bake 10 minutes or until bubbly and lightly browned.

MAKES 6 TO 8 SERVINGS

Calories 360, Total Fat 15g, Saturated Fat 6g, Cholesterol 60mg, Sodium 460mg, Carbohydrates 30g, Dietary Fiber 6g, Protein 26g

MINI MEATLOAVES

3 tablespoons tomato paste

1 tablespoon balsamic vinegar

1 tablespoon olive oil

1½ cups finely chopped onion

1½ cups finely chopped mushrooms

1½ cups chopped baby spinach

1½ pounds extra lean ground sirloin

¾ cup old-fashioned oats

2 egg whites

½ teaspoon salt

½ teaspoon black pepper

1. Preheat oven to 375°F.

2. Spray 6 mini (4¼×2½-inch) loaf pans with nonstick cooking spray. Whisk tomato paste and vinegar in small bowl until smooth and well blended; set aside.

3. Heat oil in large skillet over medium heat. Add onion, mushrooms and spinach; cook and stir 8 minutes or until tender. Transfer to large bowl; let stand until cool enough to handle.

4. Add beef, oats, egg whites, salt and pepper to vegetables; mix well. Divide mixture evenly among prepared pans. Brush half of tomato mixture evenly over loaves.

5. Bake 15 minutes. Brush with remaining tomato mixture. Bake 5 minutes or until cooked through (160°F).

MAKES 6 SERVINGS

Calories 230, **Total Fat** 8g, **Saturated Fat** 3g, **Cholesterol** 60mg, **Sodium** 320mg, **Carbohydrates** 14g, **Dietary Fiber** 3g, **Protein** 26g

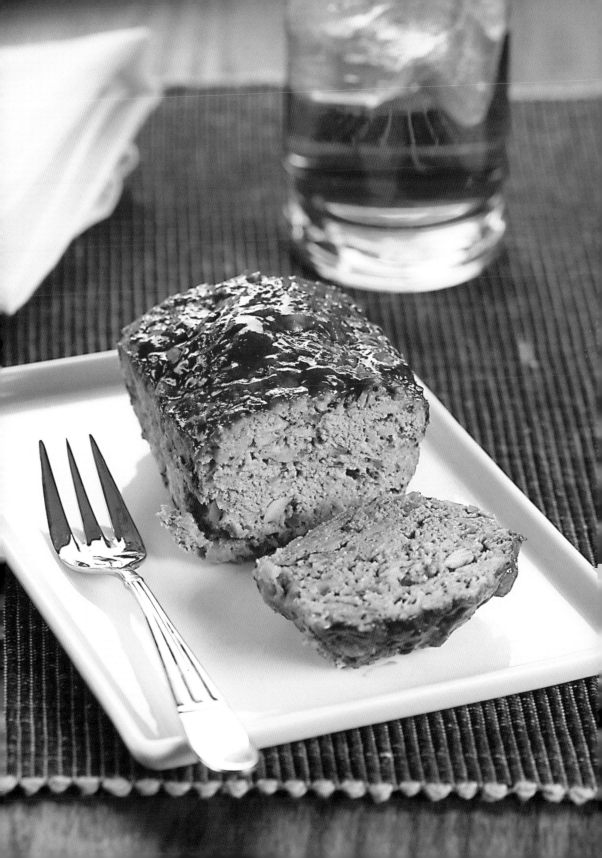

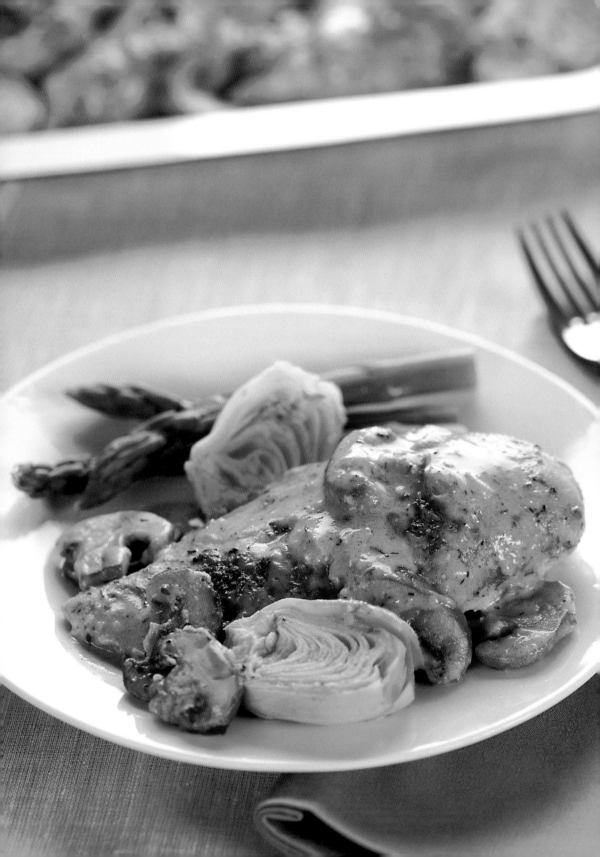

CREAMY BAKED CHICKEN WITH ARTICHOKES AND MUSHROOMS

6 boneless skinless chicken breasts (about 4 ounces each)

1½ teaspoons paprika

1½ teaspoons dried thyme

½ teaspoon salt

½ teaspoon black pepper

1 can (14 ounces) artichokes packed in water, drained

1 tablespoon butter

1 package (8 ounces) sliced cremini mushrooms

2 tablespoons all-purpose flour

¾ cup reduced-sodium chicken broth

½ cup soymilk or milk

1. Preheat oven to 375°F.

2. Place chicken in 13×9-inch baking dish. Combine paprika, thyme, salt and pepper in small bowl; mix well. Reserve 1 teaspoon seasoning mixture; set aside. Sprinkle remaining seasoning mixture evenly over chicken. Cut artichokes in half; arrange around chicken.

3. Melt butter in large saucepan over medium heat. Add mushrooms and reserved 1 teaspoon seasoning mixture; cook and stir 5 minutes or until tender. Sprinkle flour over mushrooms; cook and stir 1 minute. Stir in broth; simmer 3 minutes or until thickened. Stir in soymilk; cook 1 minute. Pour evenly over chicken and artichokes.

4. Bake 30 minutes or until chicken is no longer pink and cooked through (165°F).

MAKES 6 SERVINGS

Calories 220, **Total Fat** 5g, **Saturated Fat** 2g, **Cholesterol** 90mg, **Sodium** 750mg, **Carbohydrates** 13g, **Dietary Fiber** 2g, **Protein** 30g

SESAME-GARLIC FLANK STEAK

1 beef flank steak
(about 1¼ pounds)

2 tablespoons soy
sauce

2 tablespoons hoisin
sauce

1 tablespoon dark
sesame oil

2 cloves garlic, minced

1. Score steak lightly with sharp knife in diamond pattern on both sides; place in large resealable food storage bag. Combine soy sauce, hoisin sauce, sesame oil and garlic in small bowl; pour over steak. Seal bag; turn to coat. Marinate in refrigerator at least 2 hours or up to 24 hours, turning once.

2. Prepare grill for direct cooking. Remove steak from marinade; reserve marinade. Grill steak, covered, over medium heat 13 to 18 minutes for medium rare (145°F) to medium (160°F) or to desired doneness, turning and brushing with marinade halfway through cooking time. Discard remaining marinade.

3. Transfer steak to cutting board; carve across the grain into thin slices.

MAKES 4 SERVINGS

Calories 250, Total Fat 12g, Saturated Fat 3g, Cholesterol 90mg, Sodium 790mg, Carbohydrates 4g, Dietary Fiber 0g, Protein 31g

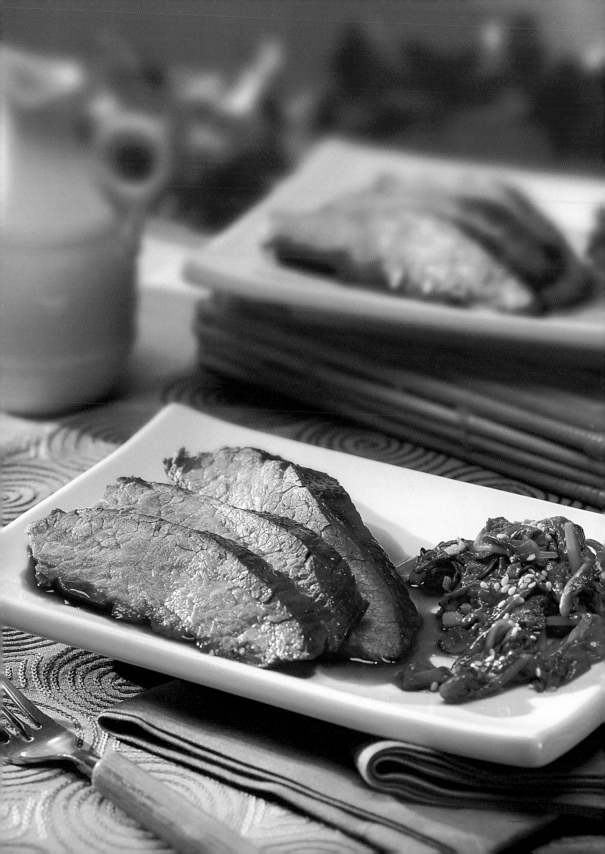

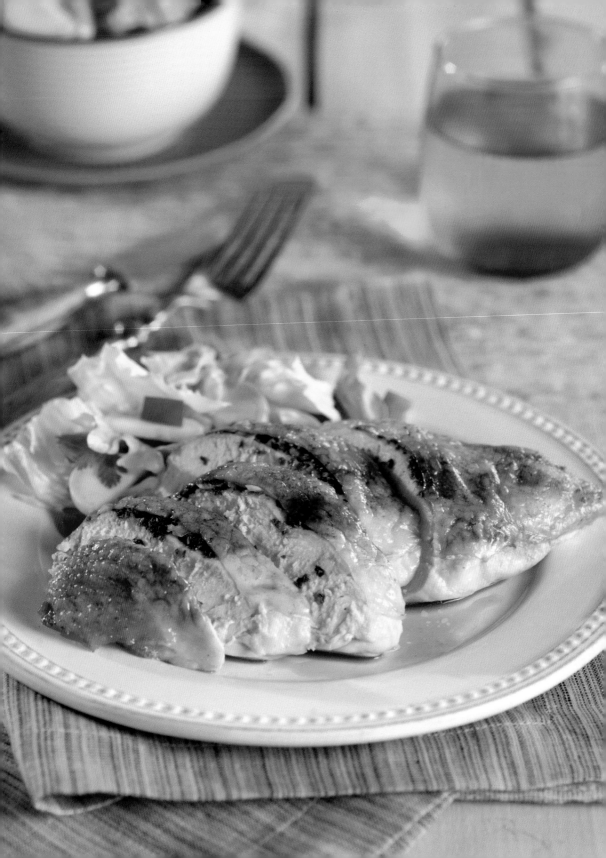

CILANTRO-STUFFED CHICKEN BREASTS

2 cloves garlic
1 cup packed fresh
   cilantro leaves
1 tablespoon plus
   2 teaspoons soy
   sauce, divided
1 tablespoon peanut or
   vegetable oil
4 boneless chicken
   breasts (about
   4 ounces each)
1 tablespoon dark
   sesame oil

1. Preheat oven to 350°F. Line shallow baking pan with foil; place rack in pan.

2. Mince garlic in blender or food processor. Add cilantro; process until finely chopped. Add 2 teaspoons soy sauce and peanut oil; process until paste forms.

3. With rubber spatula or fingers, spread about 1 tablespoon cilantro mixture evenly under skin of each chicken breast half, taking care not to puncture skin.

4. Place chicken on rack in prepared pan. Combine remaining 1 tablespoon soy sauce and sesame oil in small bowl. Brush half of mixture evenly over chicken.

5. Bake 25 minutes; brush remaining soy sauce mixture evenly over chicken. Bake 10 minutes or until cooked through (165°F).

MAKES 4 SERVINGS

Calories 240, Total Fat 16g, Saturated Fat 3g, Cholesterol 65mg, Sodium 410mg, Carbohydrates 1g, Dietary Fiber 0g, Protein 21g

GREEK CHICKEN BURGERS WITH CUCUMBER YOGURT SAUCE

½ cup plus 2 tablespoons plain nonfat Greek yogurt

½ medium cucumber, peeled, seeded and finely chopped

Juice of ½ lemon

3 cloves garlic, minced, divided

2 teaspoons finely chopped fresh mint *or* ½ teaspoon dried mint

⅛ teaspoon salt

⅛ teaspoon ground white pepper

1 pound ground chicken breast

3 ounces reduced-fat crumbled feta cheese

4 large kalamata olives, rinsed, patted dry and minced

1 egg

½ to 1 teaspoon dried oregano

¼ teaspoon black pepper

Mixed baby lettuce (optional)

1. Combine yogurt, cucumber, lemon juice, 2 cloves garlic, mint, salt and white pepper in medium bowl; mix well. Cover and refrigerate until ready to serve.

2. Combine chicken, cheese, olives, egg, oregano, black pepper and remaining 1 clove garlic in large bowl; mix well. Shape mixture into four patties.

3. Spray grill pan with nonstick cooking spray; heat over medium-high heat. Grill patties 5 to 7 minutes per side or until cooked through (165°F).

4. Serve burgers with sauce and mixed greens, if desired.

MAKES 4 SERVINGS

Calories 260, **Total Fat** 14g, **Saturated Fat** 5g, **Cholesterol** 150mg, **Sodium** 500mg, **Carbohydrates** 4g, **Dietary Fiber** 1g, **Protein** 29g

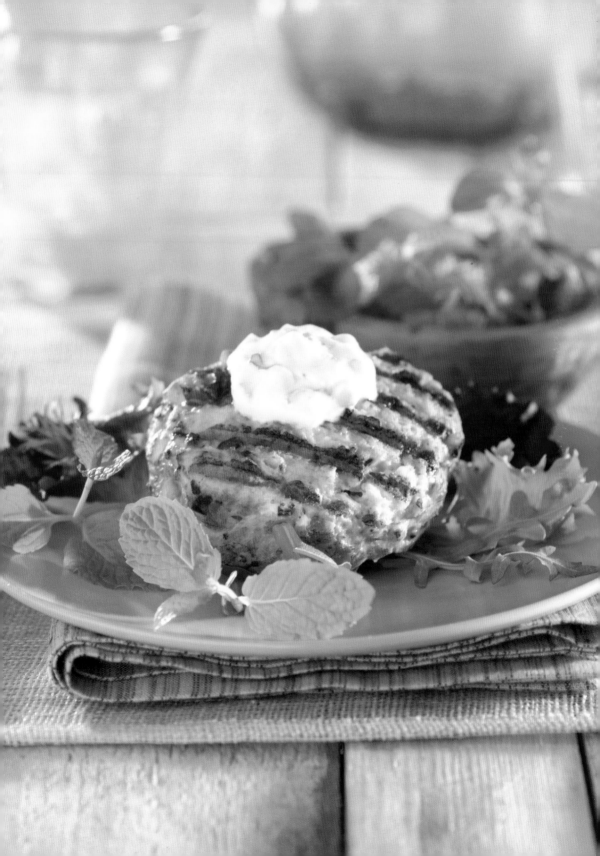

FISH & SEAFOOD

ROASTED DILL SCROD WITH ASPARAGUS

1 bunch (12 ounces) asparagus spears, ends trimmed

1 teaspoon olive oil

4 scrod or cod fillets (about 5 ounces each)

1 tablespoon lemon juice

1 teaspoon dried dill weed

½ teaspoon salt

¼ teaspoon black pepper

Paprika (optional)

1. Preheat oven to 425°F.

2. Place asparagus in 13×9-inch baking dish; drizzle with oil. Roll asparagus to coat lightly with oil; push to edges of dish, stacking asparagus into two layers.

3. Arrange fish fillets in center of dish; drizzle with lemon juice. Sprinkle dill, salt and pepper over fish and asparagus. Sprinkle with paprika, if desired.

4. Roast 15 to 17 minutes or until asparagus is crisp-tender and fish is opaque in center and begins to flake when tested with fork.

MAKES 4 SERVINGS

Calories 147, Total Fat 2g, Saturated Fat 1g, Cholesterol 61mg, Sodium 379mg, Carbohydrates 4g, Dietary Fiber 2g, Protein 27g

SEARED SCALLOPS OVER GARLIC-LEMON SPINACH

1 pound sea scallops
   (approximately 12)

¼ teaspoon salt

⅛ teaspoon black
   pepper

1 tablespoon olive oil

1 shallot, minced

2 cloves garlic, minced

1 package (6 ounces)
   baby spinach

1 tablespoon fresh
   lemon juice

   Lemon wedges
   (optional)

1. Pat scallops dry; sprinkle one side with salt and pepper. Heat oil in large nonstick skillet over medium-high heat. Add scallops; cook 2 to 3 minutes per side or until golden. Transfer to large plate; keep warm.

2. Add shallot and garlic to skillet; cook and stir 30 seconds or until fragrant. Add spinach; cook 2 minutes or until spinach just begins to wilt, stirring occasionally. Remove from heat; stir in lemon juice.

3. Serve scallops over spinach. Garnish with lemon wedges.

MAKES 4 SERVINGS

Calories 172, Total Fat 5g, Saturated Fat 1g, Cholesterol 60mg, Sodium 480mg, Carbohydrates 3g, Dietary Fiber 1g, Protein 28g

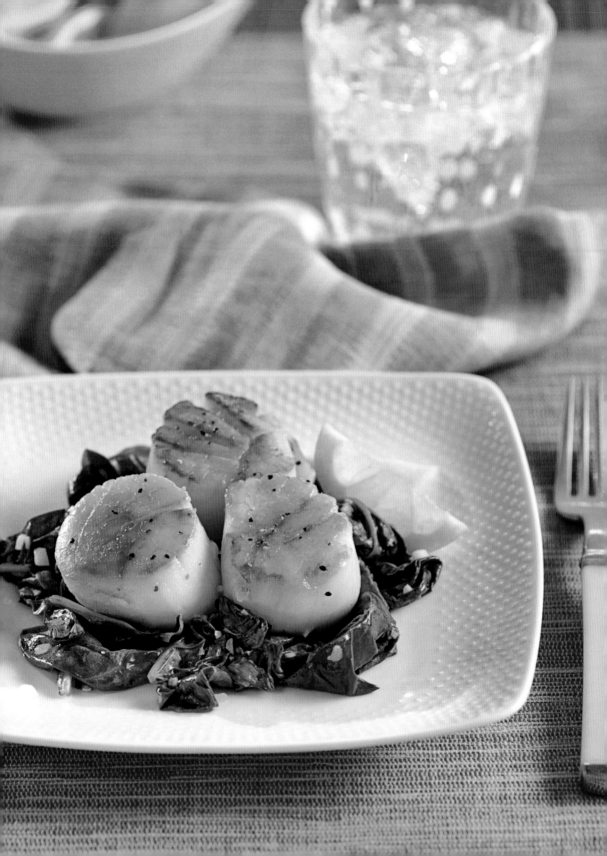

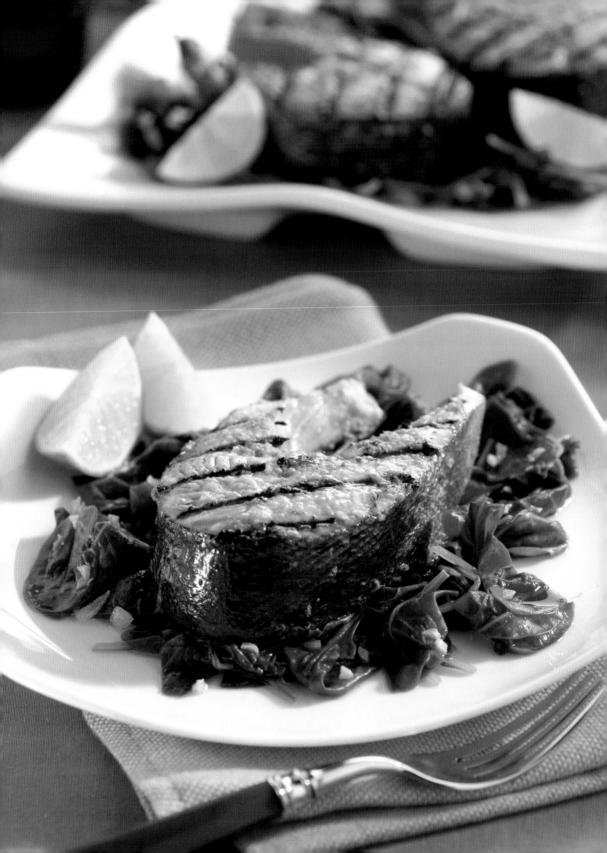

GRILLED FIVE-SPICE FISH WITH GARLIC SPINACH

1½ teaspoons grated lime peel

3 tablespoons fresh lime juice

4 teaspoons minced fresh ginger

½ to 1 teaspoon Chinese five-spice powder

½ teaspoon sugar

½ teaspoon salt

⅛ teaspoon black pepper

2 teaspoons vegetable oil, divided

1 pound salmon steaks

8 ounces fresh baby spinach leaves (about 8 cups lightly packed)

2 cloves garlic, minced

1. Combine lime peel, lime juice, ginger, five-spice powder, sugar, salt, pepper and 1 teaspoon oil in 2-quart dish. Add salmon; turn to coat. Cover and refrigerate 2 to 3 hours.

2. Combine spinach, garlic and remaining 1 teaspoon oil in 3-quart microwavable dish; toss. Cover and microwave on HIGH 2 minutes or until spinach is wilted. Drain; keep warm.

3. Meanwhile, oil grid and prepare grill for direct cooking over medium-high heat.

4. Place salmon on grid; brush with marinade. Grill, covered, 4 minutes. Turn and brush with marinade; grill 4 minutes or until fish just begins to flake when tested with fork. Discard remaining marinade.

5. Divide spinach among four serving plates; top with salmon.

MAKES 4 SERVINGS

Calories 241, **Total Fat** 15g, **Saturated Fat** 3g, **Cholesterol** 66mg, **Sodium** 426mg, **Carbohydrates** 3g, **Dietary Fiber** 1g, **Protein** 24g

BLACKENED SHRIMP
WITH TOMATOES

1½ teaspoons paprika

1 teaspoon dried Italian seasoning

½ teaspoon garlic powder

¼ teaspoon black pepper

8 ounces small raw shrimp (about 24), peeled

1 tablespoon canola oil

½ cup sliced red onion, separated into rings

1½ cups halved grape tomatoes

Lime wedges (optional)

1. Combine paprika, Italian seasoning, garlic powder and pepper in large resealable food storage bag. Add shrimp, seal bag and shake to coat.

2. Heat oil in large nonstick skillet over medium-high heat. Add shrimp; cook 4 minutes or until shrimp are pink and opaque, turning occasionally. Add onion and tomatoes; cook and stir 1 minute or until tomatoes are hot and onion is slightly wilted. Serve with lime wedges, if desired.

MAKES 4 SERVINGS

Calories 112, **Total Fat** 5g, **Saturated Fat** 1g, **Cholesterol** 86mg, **Sodium** 88mg, **Carbohydrates** 5g, **Dietary Fiber** 1g, **Protein** 13g

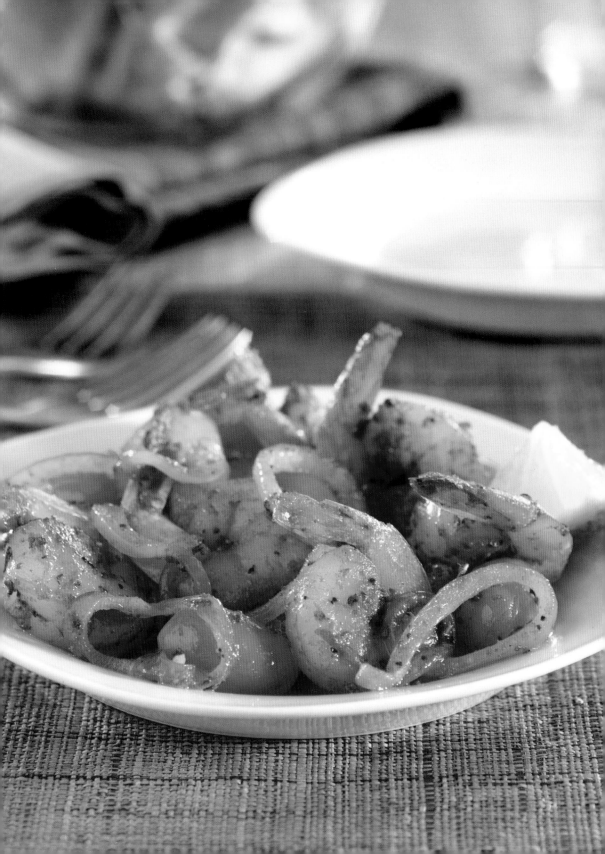

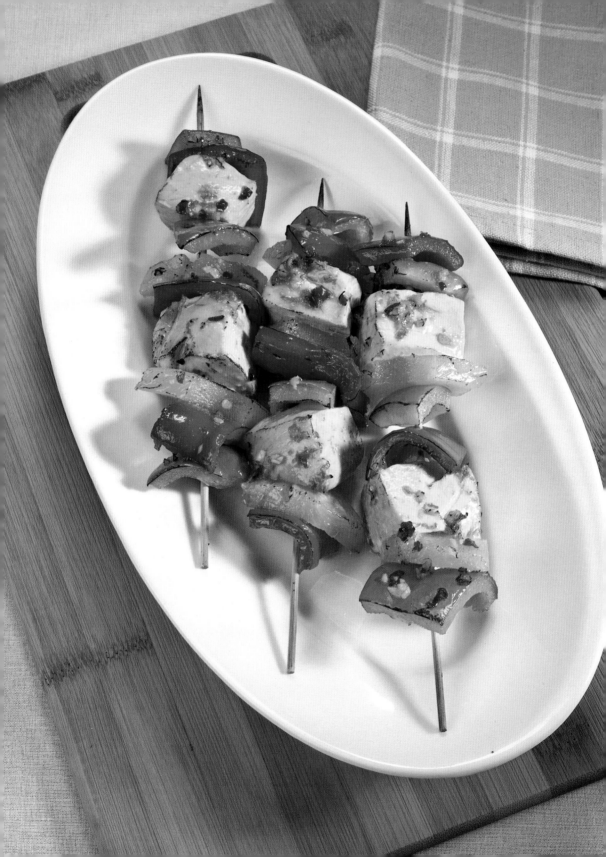

ISLAND MAHIMAHI KABOBS

1 pound mahimahi fillets, cut into 1-inch cubes

27 canned pineapple chunks in juice, drained and 2 tablespoons juice reserved

1 medium red bell pepper, cut into 1-inch chunks

1 medium green bell pepper, cut into 1-inch chunks

2 teaspoons vegetable oil

2 teaspoons grated fresh ginger

1 teaspoon reduced-sodium soy sauce

Grated peel and juice of 1 lime

¼ teaspoon red pepper flakes

1. Soak bamboo skewers in water 30 minutes to prevent scorching. Thread fish, pineapple and bell peppers alternately onto skewers.

2. Combine reserved pineapple juice, oil, ginger, soy sauce, lime peel, lime juice and red pepper flakes in small bowl. Brush half of marinade over kabobs.

3. Preheat grill or indoor grill pan to medium-high heat. Grill kabobs 3 minutes per side or until fish is opaque in center, brushing with remaining marinade.

MAKES 3 SERVINGS

Calories 226, Total Fat 4g, Saturated Fat 1g, Cholesterol 110mg, Sodium 206mg, Carbohydrates 16g, Dietary Fiber 3g, Protein 29g

GINGER-SCENTED HALIBUT

¼ cup orange juice

2 tablespoons reduced-sodium soy sauce

1½ teaspoons unseasoned rice vinegar or white wine vinegar

1 teaspoon dark sesame oil

4 halibut steaks (about ¾ inch thick)

1 tablespoon slivered fresh ginger

2 green onions, finely chopped (optional)

1. For sauce, combine orange juice, soy sauce and vinegar in small saucepan; bring to a boil. Remove from heat; stir in oil.

2. Place lightly oiled wire steaming rack or bamboo steamer in wok or large saucepan. Add water to ½ inch below rack (water should not touch rack). Cover wok; bring water to a boil over high heat. Carefully place halibut on rack in single layer; sprinkle evenly with ginger. Cover and steam 8 to 10 minutes or until halibut flakes easily when tested with fork.

3. Transfer halibut to serving plates with slotted spoon. Serve with sauce and green onions, if desired.

MAKES 4 SERVINGS

Calories 150, **Total Fat** 5g, **Saturated Fat** 1g, **Cholesterol** 85mg, **Sodium** 420mg, **Carbohydrates** 3g, Dietary Fiber 0g, **Protein** 26g

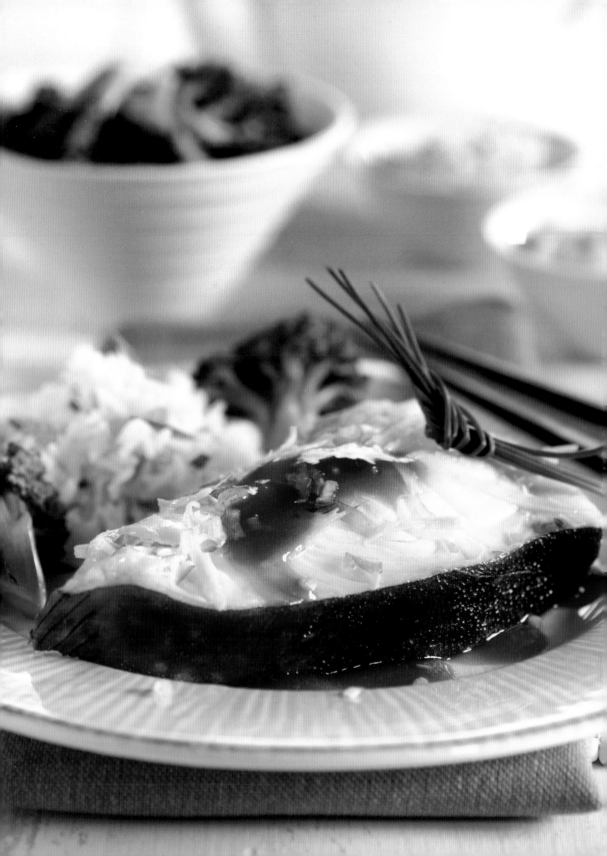

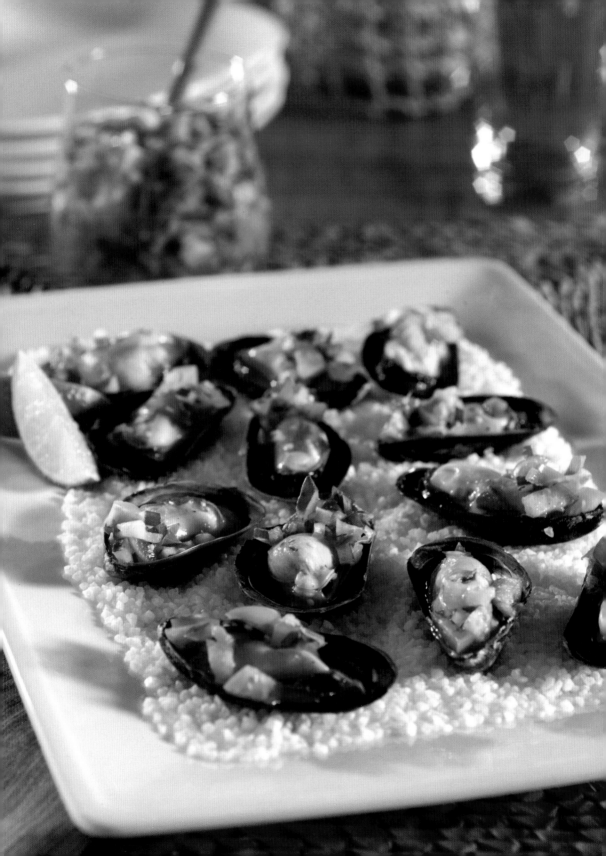

MARINATED MUSSELS

½ cup Tomatillo Salsa (recipe follows)

36 mussels or small hard-shell clams

Boiling water

1 tablespoon olive oil

1 tablespoon lime juice

Salt

1. Prepare Tomatillo Salsa.

2. Scrub mussels under cold running water with stiff brush; discard any with open shells or with shells that do not close when tapped. Arrange half of mussels in large skillet; pour in boiling water to depth of about ½ inch. Cover and simmer over medium heat 5 to 8 minutes or until shells open. As their shells open, remove mussels with slotted spoon; set aside to cool. Discard any unopened mussels. Repeat with remaining mussels.

3. Remove mussels from shells with small knife. Separate shells; save half. Cover shells and refrigerate. Combine salsa, oil and lime juice in large bowl. Add mussels; stir to coat. Season with salt to taste. Cover and refrigerate up to 24 hours.

4. Remove mussels from salsa; place one in each shell. Arrange on platter. Spoon salsa over mussels.

MAKES 6 TO 8 SERVINGS

TOMATILLO SALSA

1 pound tomatillos (about 12 large) *or* 1 can (13 ounces) tomatillos

½ cup finely chopped red onion

¼ cup coarsely chopped fresh cilantro

2 jalapeño or serrano peppers, seeded and minced

1 tablespoon lime juice

1 teaspoon olive oil

½ teaspoon salt

1. For fresh tomatillos, remove papery husks, wash and finely chop. For canned tomatillos, drain and coarsely chop.

2. Combine tomatillos, onion, cilantro, jalapeño peppers, lime juice, oil and salt medium bowl. Cover and refrigerate 1 hour or up to 3 days.

Calories 350, **Total Fat** 12g, **Saturated Fat** 2g, **Cholesterol** 95mg, **Sodium** 830mg, **Carbohydrates** 20g, **Dietary Fiber** 2g, **Protein** 41g

GRILLED TILAPIA WITH ZESTY MUSTARD SAUCE

2 tablespoons olive oil

1 teaspoon Dijon mustard

½ teaspoon grated lemon peel

½ teaspoon Worcestershire sauce

½ teaspoon salt, divided

¼ teaspoon black pepper

4 tilapia fillets or other mild white fish (about 4 ounces each)

1½ teaspoons paprika

½ lemon, quartered

2 tablespoons minced fresh parsley (optional)

1. Prepare grill for direct cooking over high heat.

2. Whisk oil, mustard, lemon peel, Worcestershire sauce, ¼ teaspoon salt and pepper in small bowl until well blended. Set aside.

3. Rinse fish and pat dry with paper towels. Sprinkle both sides of fish with paprika and remaining ¼ teaspoon salt. Lightly spray grill basket with nonstick cooking spray. Place fish in basket.

4. Grill, covered, 3 minutes. Turn and grill, covered, 2 to 3 minutes or until fish flakes easily when tested with fork. Transfer to platter.

5. Squeeze one lemon wedge over each fillet. Spread mustard sauce evenly over fish. Sprinkle with parsley, if desired.

MAKES 4 SERVINGS

Calories 170, Total Fat 9g, Saturated Fat 1g, Cholesterol 55mg, Sodium 390mg, Carbohydrates 1g, Dietary Fiber 0g, Protein 23g

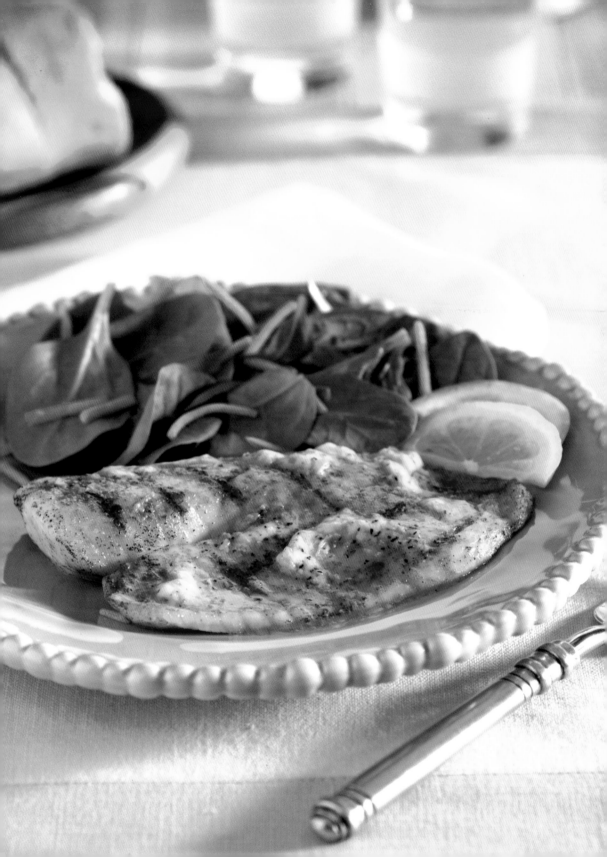

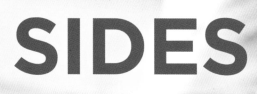

SIDES

MEDITERRANEAN-STYLE ROASTED VEGETABLES

1½ pounds red potatoes, cut into ½-inch chunks

1 tablespoon plus 1½ teaspoons olive oil, divided

1 red bell pepper, cut into ½-inch pieces

1 yellow or orange bell pepper, cut into ½-inch pieces

1 small red onion, cut into ½-inch wedges

2 cloves garlic, minced

½ teaspoon salt

¼ teaspoon black pepper

1 tablespoon balsamic vinegar

¼ cup chopped fresh basil

1. Preheat oven to 425°F. Spray large roasting pan with nonstick cooking spray.

2. Place potatoes in prepared pan. Drizzle with 1 tablespoon oil; toss to coat evenly. Roast 10 minutes.

3. Add bell peppers and onion to pan. Drizzle with remaining 1½ teaspoons oil. Sprinkle with garlic, salt and black pepper; toss to coat evenly.

4. Roast 18 to 20 minutes or until vegetables are browned and tender, stirring once.

5. Transfer vegetables to large serving dish. Drizzle vinegar over vegetables; toss to coat. Gently stir in basil. Serve warm or at room temperature.

MAKES 6 SERVINGS

Calories 170, **Total Fat** 4g, **Saturated Fat** 1g, **Cholesterol** 0mg, **Sodium** 185mg, **Carbohydrates** 33g, **Dietary Fiber** 1g, **Protein** 3g

WILD MUSHROOM QUINOA STUFFING

1 cup uncooked quinoa

2 tablespoons olive oil, divided

2 cups vegetable broth

1 teaspoon poultry seasoning

½ teaspoon salt

1 small onion, diced

8 ounces cremini mushrooms, sliced

8 ounces shiitake mushrooms, stemmed and sliced

½ cup diced celery

2 tablespoons chopped fresh parsley (optional)

1. Place quinoa in fine-mesh strainer; rinse well under cold running water.

2. Heat 1 tablespoon oil in medium saucepan over medium-high heat. Add quinoa; stir until evenly coated. Stir in broth, poultry seasoning and salt. Bring to a boil. Reduce heat to low; cover and simmer 15 to 20 minutes or until quinoa is tender and broth is absorbed. Remove from heat.

3. Meanwhile, heat remaining 1 tablespoon oil in large skillet over medium heat. Add onion, mushrooms and celery; cook and stir 8 to 10 minutes or until vegetables are tender.

4. Combine quinoa and vegetables in large bowl. Sprinkle with parsley, if desired.

MAKES 6 SERVINGS

Tip: *Serve this tasty side any time, or use it as a stuffing for turkey or chicken.*

Calories 181, Total Fat 6g, Saturated Fat 1g, Cholesterol 0mg, Sodium 392mg, Carbohydrates 25g, Dietary Fiber 4g, Protein 7g

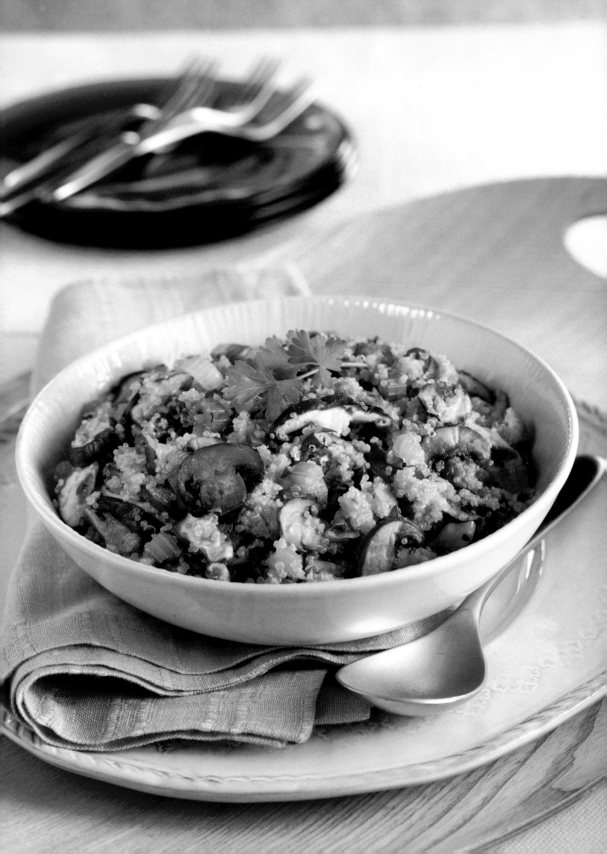

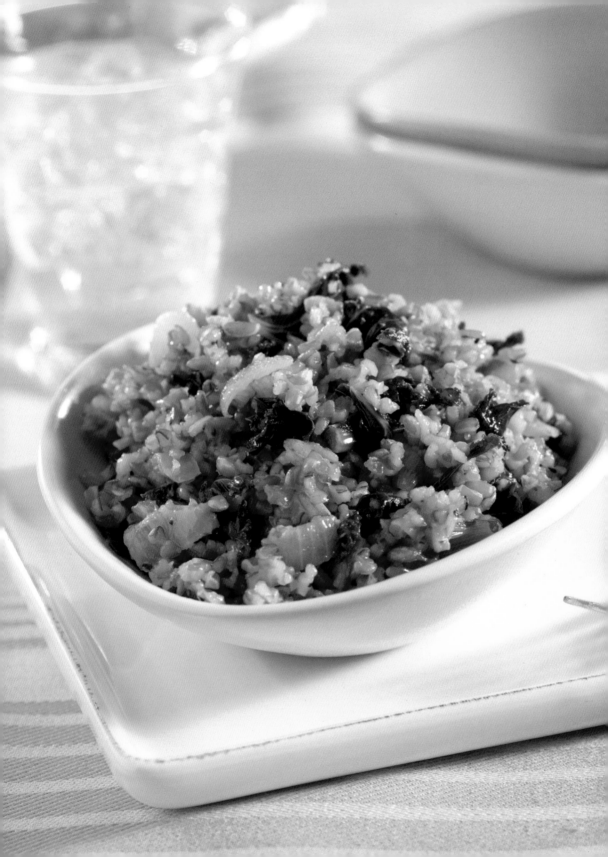

BULGUR PILAF WITH CARAMELIZED ONIONS AND KALE

1 tablespoon olive oil

1 onion, thinly sliced

1 clove garlic, minced

2 cups chopped kale

2 cups vegetable broth

¾ cup uncooked medium grain bulgur

½ teaspoon salt

¼ teaspoon black pepper

1. Heat oil in large nonstick skillet over medium heat. Add onion; cook 10 minutes or until softened and lightly browned, stirring frequently. Add garlic; cook and stir 1 minute. Add kale; cook and stir about 1 minute or until kale is wilted.

2. Stir in broth, bulgur, salt and pepper. Bring to a boil. Reduce heat; cover and simmer 12 minutes or until liquid is absorbed and bulgur is tender.

MAKES 6 SERVINGS

Calories 165, **Total Fat** 4g, **Saturated Fat** 1g, **Cholesterol** 0mg, **Sodium** 540mg, **Carbohydrates** 29g, **Dietary Fiber** 6g, **Protein** 5g

BUTTERNUT SQUASH OVEN CHIPS

Lime Yogurt Dip
  (recipe follows)
½ teaspoon garlic
  powder
¼ teaspoon salt
¼ teaspoon ground
  red pepper
1 butternut squash
  (about 2½ pounds)
2 teaspoons
  vegetable oil

1. Preheat oven to 425°F. Prepare Lime Yogurt Dip. Combine garlic powder, salt and red pepper in small bowl.

2. Peel and seed squash. Cut in half lengthwise; cut into thin slices. Spread squash on baking sheet. Drizzle with oil and sprinkle with seasoning mix; gently toss to coat. Arrange in single layer.

3. Bake 20 to 25 minutes or until squash is browned and crisp, turning occasionally.

MAKES 4 SERVINGS

Lime Yogurt Dip: *Combine ¼ cup reduced-fat mayonnaise, ¼ cup reduced-fat Greek yogurt, 1 teaspoon lime juice and ¼ teaspoon grated lime peel in small bowl. Refrigerate until ready to serve.*

Tip: *You can also use a spiralizer to cut the squash. Peel and seed the squash and cut it crosswise into 3-inch pieces. Spiral the squash pieces with the thick spiral blade and then cut in half to form semicircles.*

Calories 190, Total Fat 8g, Saturated Fat 1g, Cholesterol 5mg, Sodium 260mg, Carbohydrates 32g, Dietary Fiber 5g, Protein 4g

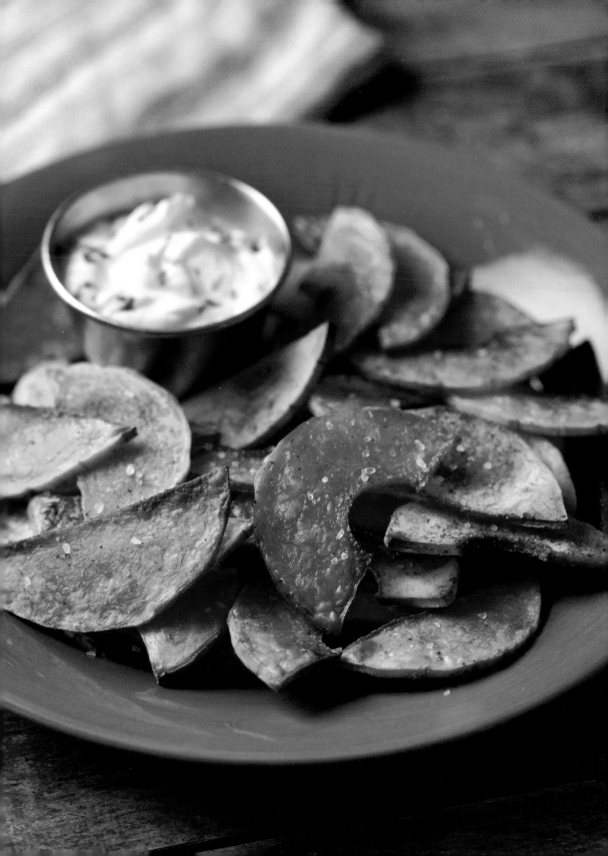

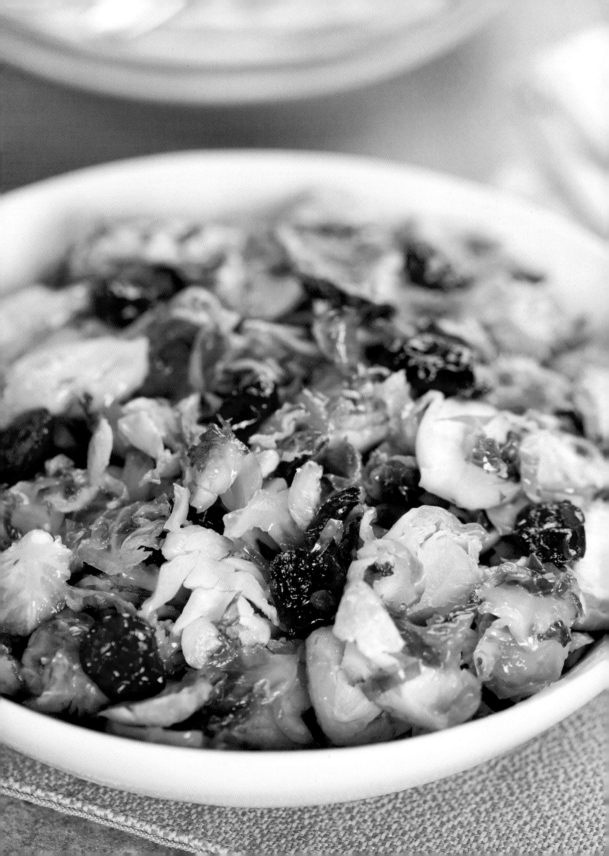

CARAMELIZED BRUSSELS SPROUTS WITH CRANBERRIES

1 tablespoon vegetable oil

1 pound Brussels sprouts, ends trimmed and discarded, thinly sliced

¼ cup dried cranberries

2 teaspoons packed brown sugar

¼ teaspoon salt

1. Heat oil in large skillet over medium-high heat. Add Brussels sprouts; cook and stir 10 minutes or until crisp-tender and beginning to brown.

2. Add cranberries, brown sugar and salt; cook and stir 5 minutes or until browned.

MAKES 4 SERVINGS

Calories 105, Total Fat 4g, Saturated Fat 1g, Cholesterol 0mg, Sodium 317mg, Carbohydrates 17g, Dietary Fiber 4g, Protein 3g

MEDITERRANEAN VEGETABLE BAKE

1 small red onion

1 medium zucchini

1 small yellow squash

2 tomatoes, sliced

1 small eggplant

1 large portobello mushroom, sliced

2 cloves garlic, finely chopped

3 tablespoons olive oil

2 teaspoons chopped fresh rosemary leaves

⅔ cup dry white wine

Salt and black pepper

1. Preheat oven to 350°F. Grease shallow casserole or 13×9-inch baking dish.

2. Using spiralizer, spiral red onion, zucchini and yellow squash with thick spiral blade. Arrange spiraled vegetables, tomatoes, eggplant and mushroom alternately in prepared baking dish. Sprinkle evenly with garlic. Combine oil and rosemary in small bowl; drizzle over vegetables. Pour wine over vegetables; season with salt and pepper. Cover loosely with foil.

3. Bake 20 minutes. Uncover; bake 10 to 15 minutes or until vegetables are tender.

MAKES 4 TO 6 SERVINGS

Tip: *If you don't have a spiralizer, thinly slice the onion, zucchini and squash and layer them in the baking dish with the tomatoes, eggplant and mushrooms*

Calories 230, Total Fat 1.5g, Saturated Fat 0g, Cholesterol 0mg, Sodium 20mg, Carbohydrates 25g, Dietary Fiber 5g, Protein 4g

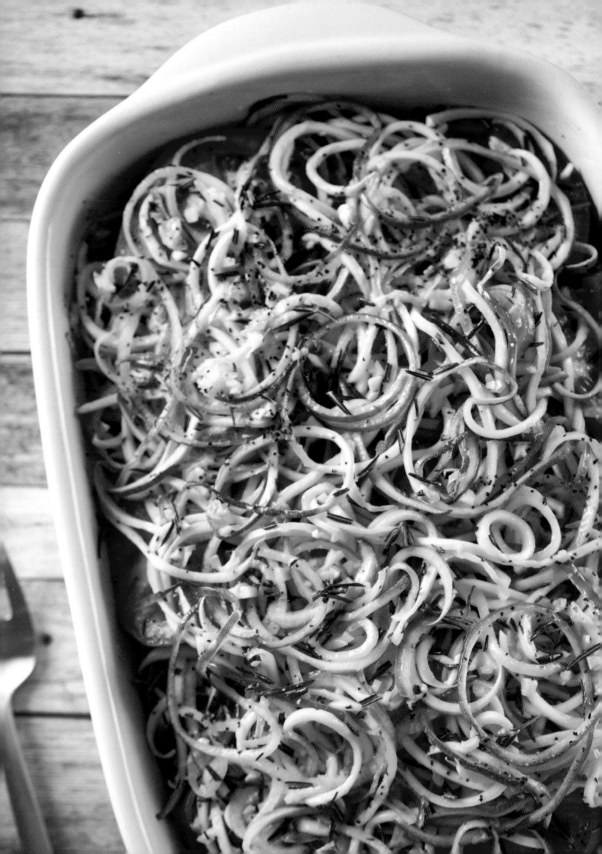

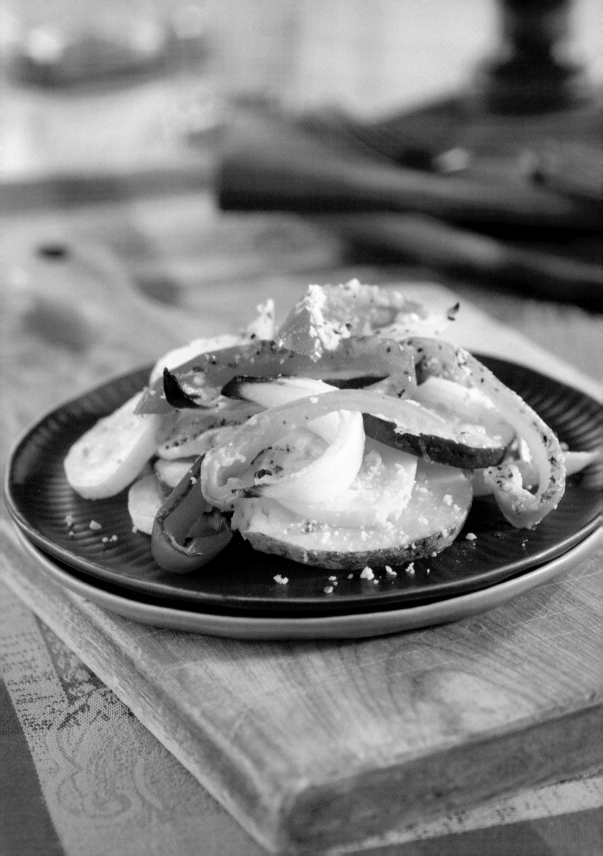

PEPPER AND SQUASH GRATIN

1 russet potato
  (12 ounces)

8 ounces yellow
  summer squash,
  thinly sliced

8 ounces zucchini,
  thinly sliced

1½ cups red and/or
  green bell pepper
  strips

½ cup sliced onion

1 teaspoon dried
  oregano

½ teaspoon salt

⅛ teaspoon black
  pepper (optional)

½ cup grated Parmesan
  cheese

1 tablespoon butter,
  cut into 8 pieces

1. Preheat oven to 375°F. Spray 12×8-inch baking dish with nonstick cooking spray.

2. Pierce potato several times with fork. Microwave on HIGH 3 minutes. Cut potato into thin slices.

3. Layer half of potato slices, yellow squash, zucchini, bell pepper, onion, oregano, salt, black pepper, if desired, and cheese in prepared baking dish. Repeat layers. Dot with butter.

4. Cover tightly with foil; bake 25 minutes or until vegetables are just tender. Remove foil; bake 10 minutes more or until lightly browned.

MAKES 8 SERVINGS

Calories 106, **Total Fat** 3g, **Saturated Fat** 2g, **Cholesterol** 8mg, **Sodium** 267mg, **Carbohydrates** 15g, **Dietary Fiber** 2g, **Protein** 4g

QUINOA AND ROASTED CORN

1 cup uncooked quinoa

2 cups water

½ teaspoon salt

4 ears corn *or* 2 cups frozen corn

¼ cup plus 1 tablespoon vegetable oil, divided

1 cup chopped green onions, divided

1 teaspoon coarse salt

1 cup quartered grape tomatoes or chopped plum tomatoes

1 cup canned black beans, rinsed and drained

Juice of 1 lime (about 2 tablespoons)

¼ teaspoon grated lime peel

¼ teaspoon sugar

¼ teaspoon ground cumin

¼ teaspoon black pepper

1. Place quinoa in fine-mesh strainer; rinse well under cold running water. Combine quinoa, water and salt in medium saucepan; bring to a boil over high heat. Reduce heat to low; cover and simmer 15 to 18 minutes or until quinoa is tender and water is absorbed. Transfer to large bowl.

2. Meanwhile, remove husks and silk from corn; cut kernels off cobs. Heat ¼ cup oil in large skillet over medium-high heat. Add corn; cook 10 to 12 minutes or until tender and lightly browned, stirring occasionally. Stir in ⅔ cup green onions and coarse salt; cook and stir 2 minutes. Add corn mixture to quinoa. Gently stir in tomatoes and black beans.

3. Combine lime juice, lime peel, sugar, cumin and black pepper in small bowl. Whisk in remaining 1 tablespoon oil until blended. Pour over quinoa mixture; toss lightly to coat. Sprinkle with remaining ⅓ cup green onions. Serve warm or cold.

MAKES 8 SERVINGS

Calories 220, Total Fat 10g, Saturated Fat 2g, Cholesterol 0mg, Sodium 540mg, Carbohydrates 27g, Dietary Fiber 4g, Protein 6g

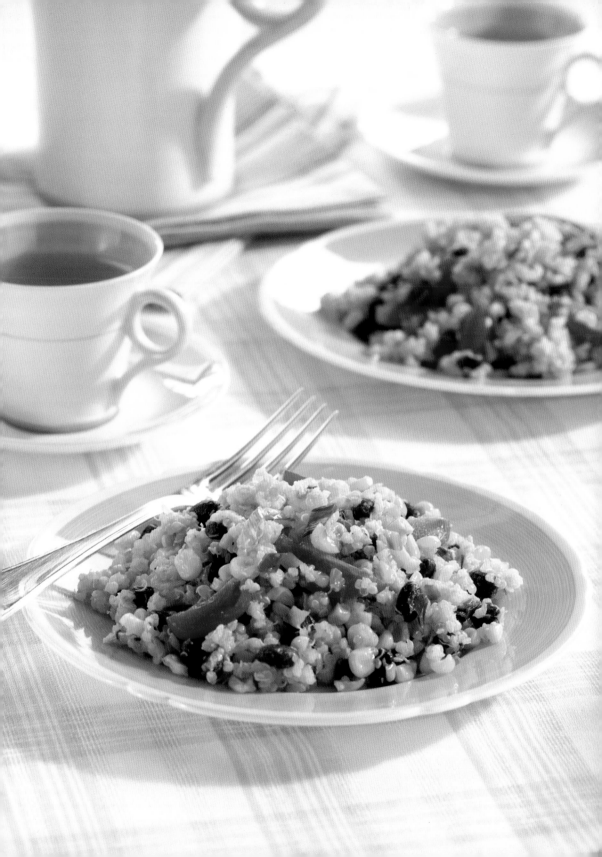

SMOOTHIES

<< SWEET GREEN SUPREME

2 cups seedless green
  grapes
½ frozen banana
½ cup baby kale
½ cup ice cubes

Combine grapes, banana, kale and ice in blender; blend until smooth. Serve immediately.

MAKES 2 SERVINGS

Calories 130, Total Fat 0g, Saturated Fat 0g, Cholesterol 0mg, Sodium 0mg, Carbohydrates 37g, Dietary Fiber 3g, Protein 2g

SUPERFOODS SMOOTHIE

½ cup apple juice
1 cup packed stemmed
  kale
1 cup baby spinach
1 banana
1 cup ice cubes

Combine apple juice, kale, spinach, banana and ice in blender; blend until smooth.

MAKES 1 SERVING

Calories 155, Total Fat 1g, Saturated Fat 0g, Cholesterol 0mg, Sodium 59mg, Carbohydrates 37g, Dietary Fiber 5g, Protein 4g

STRAWBERRY CLEMENTINE SMOOTHIE >>

⅓ cup water

2 cups frozen strawberries, slightly thawed

1 frozen banana

2 clementines, peeled

Combine water, strawberries, banana and clemetines in blender; blend until smooth. Serve immediately.

MAKES 2 SERVINGS

Calories 140, Total Fat 0g, Saturated Fat 0g, Cholesterol 0mg, Sodium 0mg, Carbohydrates 35g, Dietary Fiber 6g, Protein 2g

STRAWBERRY APPLE SMOOTHIE

¾ cup water

1 sweet red apple, seeded and cut into chunks

1 clementine, peeled

1 cup frozen strawberries

1 tablespoon lemon juice

Combine water, apple, clementine, strawberries and lemon juice in blender; blend until smooth. Serve immediately.

MAKES 2 SERVINGS

Calories 110, Total Fat 0g, Saturated Fat 0g, Cholesterol 0mg, Sodium 0mg, Carbohydrates 28g, Dietary Fiber 5g, Protein 1g

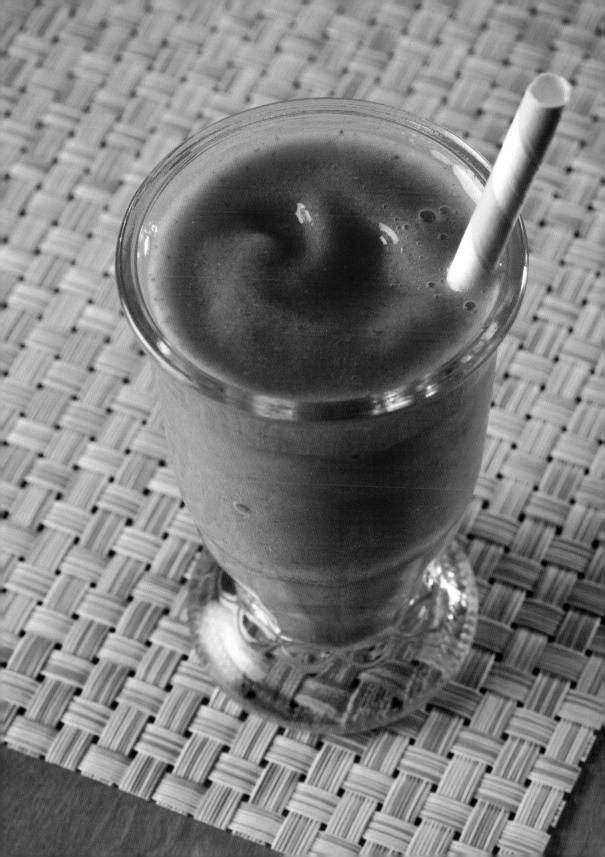

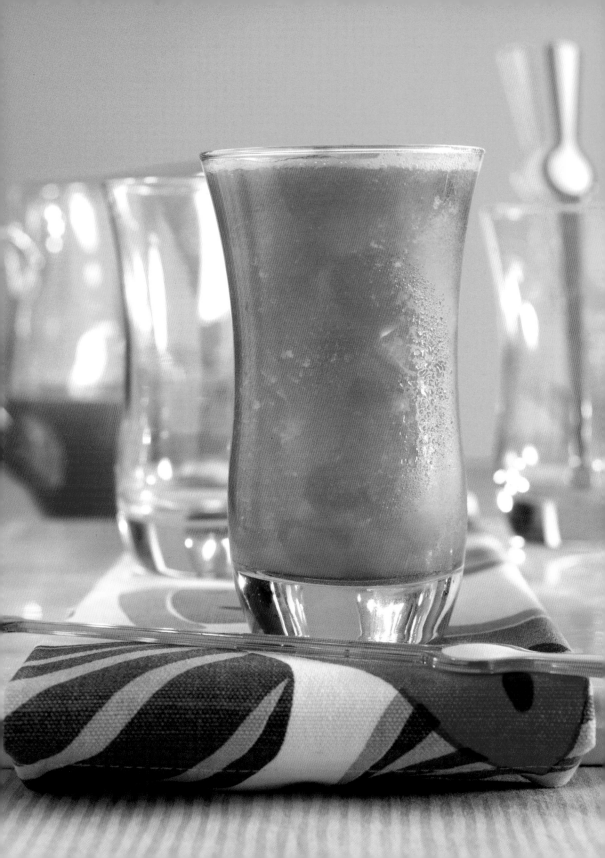

<< LEMON–LIME WATERMELON AGUA FRESCA

5 cups seedless
   watermelon cubes
½ cup ice water
   Grated peel and juice
   of 1 lemon
   Grated peel and juice
   of 1 lime

Combine watermelon, water, lemon peel and juice and lime peel and juice in blender; blend until smooth. Serve immediately over ice or refrigerate until ready to serve.

MAKES 2 SERVINGS

Calories 93, Total Fat 1g, Saturated Fat 0g, Cholesterol 0mg, Sodium 3mg, Carbohydrates 24g, Dietary Fiber 3g, Protein 2g

FROZEN WATERMELON WHIP

1 cup brewed lemon
   herbal tea, at room
   temperature
1¾ cups ice cubes
1 cup coarsely chopped
   seedless watermelon
   Lime slices (optional)

1. Combine tea, ice and watermelon in blender; blend until smooth.

2. Pour into two tall glasses. Garnish with lime. Serve immediately.

MAKES 2 SERVINGS

Calories 24, Total Fat 1g, Saturated Fat 1g, Cholesterol 0mg, Sodium 2mg, Carbohydrates 6g, Dietary Fiber 1g, Protein 1g

PINEAPPLE CRUSH >>

½ cup unsweetened coconut milk

1½ cups frozen pineapple chunks

¼ cup ice cubes

½ teaspoon vanilla

Combine coconut milk, pineapple, ice and vanilla in blender; blend until smooth. Serve immediately.

MAKES 2 SERVINGS

Calories 170, Total Fat 3g, Saturated Fat 3g, Cholesterol 0mg, Sodium 10mg, Carbohydrates 37g, Dietary Fiber 4g, Protein 3g

ISLAND DELIGHT SMOOTHIE

1 cup unsweetened almond milk

1 frozen banana

½ cup frozen mango chunks

1 tablespoon almond butter

Combine almond milk, banana, mango and almond butter in blender; blend until smooth. Serve immediately.

MAKES 2 SERVINGS

Calories 150, Total Fat 5g, Saturated Fat 0g, Cholesterol 0mg, Sodium 85mg, Carbohydrates 24g, Dietary Fiber 4g, Protein 3g

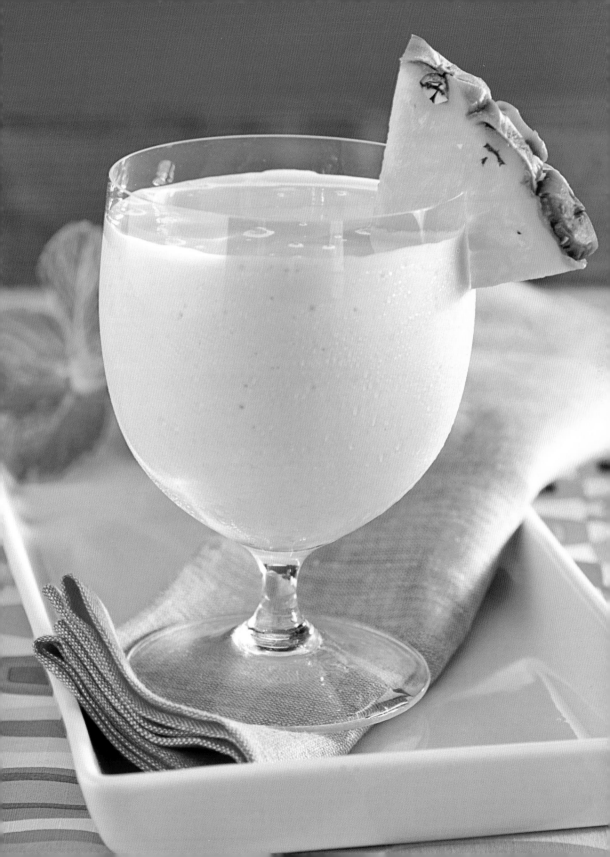

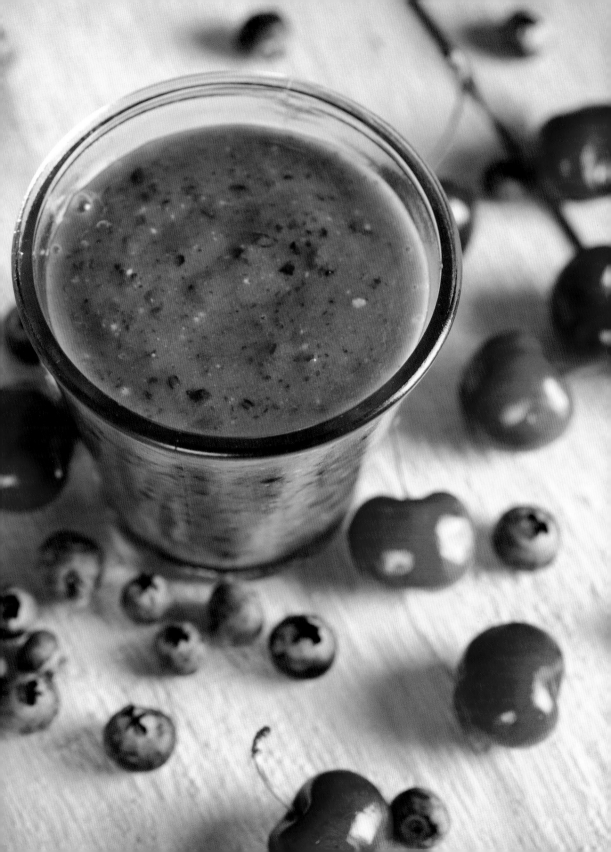

<< BLUEBERRY CHERRY BLEND

- ¾ cup water
- ¾ cup frozen blueberries
- ¾ cup frozen dark sweet cherries
- ½ avocado, pitted and peeled
- 1 tablespoon lemon juice
- 1 teaspoon ground flaxseed

Combine water, blueberries, cherries, avocado, lemon juice and flaxseed in blender; blend until smooth. Serve immediately.

MAKES 2 SERVINGS

Calories 150, Total Fat 8g, Saturated Fat 1g, Cholesterol 0mg, Sodium 0mg, Carbohydrates 20g, Dietary Fiber 6g, Protein 2g

CHERRY GREEN SMOOTHIE

- ¾ cup almond milk
- 1½ cups frozen dark sweet cherries
- ¾ cup baby spinach
- ½ frozen banana
- 1 tablespoon ground flaxseed

Combine almond milk, cherries, spinach, banana and flaxseed in blender; blend until smooth. Serve immediately.

MAKES 2 SERVINGS

Calories 140, Total Fat 2.5g, Saturated Fat 0g, Cholesterol 0mg, Sodium 75mg, Carbohydrates 28g, Dietary Fiber 5g, Protein 3g

KIWI MANGO MAGIC >>

- 1 cup water
- 2 kiwis, peeled and quartered
- ¾ cup frozen pineapple chunks
- ¾ cup frozen mango chunks
- ⅓ cup fresh mint leaves (about 3 sprigs)

Combine water, kiwis, pineapple, mango and mint in blender; blend until smooth. Serve immediately.

MAKES 2 SERVINGS

Calories 130, Total Fat 0g, Saturated Fat 0g, Cholesterol 0mg, Sodium 0mg, Carbohydrates 33g, Dietary Fiber 5g, Protein 2g

TANGY APPLE KALE SMOOTHIE

- 1 cup water
- 2 Granny Smith apples, seeded and cut into chunks
- 2 cups baby kale
- 1 frozen banana

Combine water, apples, kale and banana in blender; blend until smooth. Serve immediately.

MAKES 3 SERVINGS

Calories 100, Total Fat 0g, Saturated Fat 0g, Cholesterol 0mg, Sodium 5mg, Carbohydrates 25g, Dietary Fiber 5g, Protein 1g

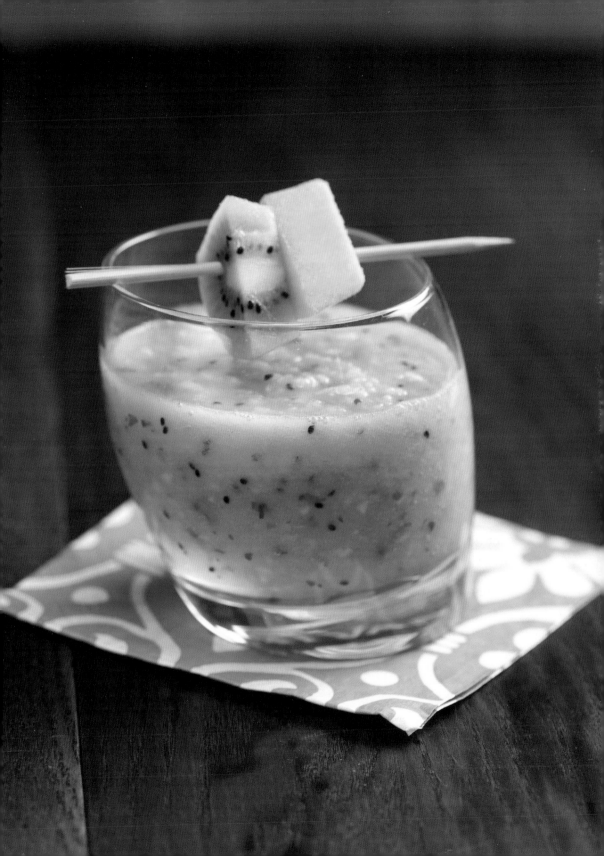

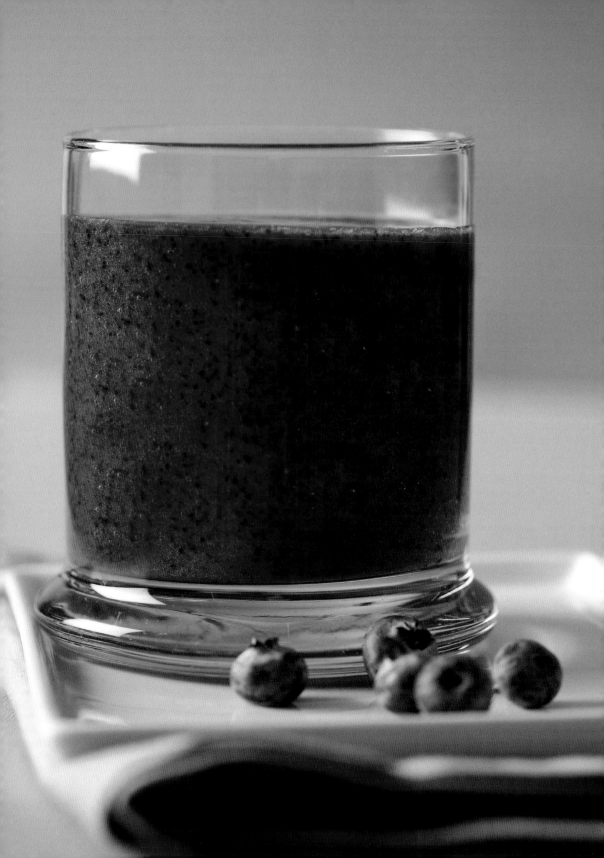

<< PURPLE PICK-ME-UP

¼ cup water
1 navel orange, peeled and seeded
1 cup frozen blueberries
4 Medjool dates, pitted

Combine water, orange, blueberries and dates in blender; blend until smooth. Serve immediately.

MAKES 2 SERVINGS

Calories 230, **Total Fat** 0.5g, **Saturated Fat** 0g, **Cholesterol** 0mg, **Sodium** 0mg, **Carbohydrates** 60g, **Dietary Fiber** 7g, **Protein** 2g

SWEET BEET TREAT

¼ cup water
2 medium carrots, cut into chunks (about 4 ounces)
1 medium beet, peeled and cut into chunks
1 large sweet red apple, seeded and cut into chunks
¼ cup ice cubes
1 tablespoon lemon juice

Combine water, carrots, beet, apple, ice and lemon juice in blender; blend until smooth. Serve immediately.

MAKES 2 SERVINGS

Calories 110, **Total Fat** 0g, **Saturated Fat** 0g, **Cholesterol** 0mg, **Sodium** 70mg, **Carbohydrates** 27g, **Dietary Fiber** 5g, **Protein** 2g

METRIC CONVERSION CHART

VOLUME MEASUREMENTS (dry)

$1/8$ teaspoon = 0.5 mL
$1/4$ teaspoon = 1 mL
$1/2$ teaspoon = 2 mL
$3/4$ teaspoon = 4 mL
1 teaspoon = 5 mL
1 tablespoon = 15 mL
2 tablespoons = 30 mL
$1/4$ cup = 60 mL
$1/3$ cup = 75 mL
$1/2$ cup = 125 mL
$2/3$ cup = 150 mL
$3/4$ cup = 175 mL
1 cup = 250 mL
2 cups = 1 pint = 500 mL
3 cups = 750 mL
4 cups = 1 quart = 1 L

VOLUME MEASUREMENTS (fluid)

1 fluid ounce (2 tablespoons) = 30 mL
4 fluid ounces ($1/2$ cup) = 125 mL
8 fluid ounces (1 cup) = 250 mL
12 fluid ounces ($1 1/2$ cups) = 375 mL
16 fluid ounces (2 cups) = 500 mL

WEIGHTS (mass)

$1/2$ ounce = 15 g
1 ounce = 30 g
3 ounces = 90 g
4 ounces = 120 g
8 ounces = 225 g
10 ounces = 285 g
12 ounces = 360 g
16 ounces = 1 pound = 450 g

DIMENSIONS

$1/16$ inch = 2 mm
$1/8$ inch = 3 mm
$1/4$ inch = 6 mm
$1/2$ inch = 1.5 cm
$3/4$ inch = 2 cm
1 inch = 2.5 cm

OVEN TEMPERATURES

250°F = 120°C
275°F = 140°C
300°F = 150°C
325°F = 160°C
350°F = 180°C
375°F = 190°C
400°F = 200°C
425°F = 220°C
450°F = 230°C

BAKING PAN SIZES

Utensil	Size in Inches/Quarts	Metric Volume	Size in Centimeters
Baking or Cake Pan (square or rectangular)	$8 \times 8 \times 2$	2 L	$20 \times 20 \times 5$
	$9 \times 9 \times 2$	2.5 L	$23 \times 23 \times 5$
	$12 \times 8 \times 2$	3 L	$30 \times 20 \times 5$
	$13 \times 9 \times 2$	3.5 L	$33 \times 23 \times 5$
Loaf Pan	$8 \times 4 \times 3$	1.5 L	$20 \times 10 \times 7$
	$9 \times 5 \times 3$	2 L	$23 \times 13 \times 7$
Round Layer Cake Pan	$8 \times 1 1/2$	1.2 L	20×4
	$9 \times 1 1/2$	1.5 L	23×4
Pie Plate	$8 \times 1 1/4$	750 mL	20×3
	$9 \times 1 1/4$	1 L	23×3
Baking Dish or Casserole	1 quart	1 L	—
	$1 1/2$ quart	1.5 L	—
	2 quart	2 L	—